University of Nottingham
at Derby Library

MRCP 1
POCKET BOOK
2

Basic Sciences, Neurology, and Psychiatry
Second Edition

Shani Esmail BSc MBChir MRCP
David W. Ray PhD MRCP
Edward Tobias MBChB MRCP PhD
Geraint Rees BM BCh MD MRCP PhD
M. Zoha MBChB MRCPsych

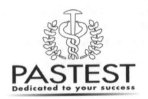

PASTEST
Dedicated to your success

© 2002 PASTEST LTD
Egerton Court, Parkgate Estate,
Knutsford, Cheshire, WA16 8DX

University of Nottingham
at Derby Library

All rights reserved. No part of this publication may be reproduced, stored in a retrieval system, or transmitted, in any form by any means, electronic, mechanical, photocopying, recording or otherwise without the prior permission of the copyright owner.

First edition 2002
Reprinted 2002, 2003
Second edition 2004

ISBN: 1 901198 89 8

A catalogue record for this book is available from the British Library.

The information contained within this book was obtained by the author from reliable sources. However, while every effort has been made to ensure its accuracy, no responsibilty for loss, damage or injury occasioned to any person acting or refraining from action as a result of information contained herein can be accepted by the publishers or author.

PasTest Revision Books and Intensive Courses

PasTest has been established in the field of postgraduate medical education since 1972, providing revision books and intensive study courses for doctors preparing for their professional examinations. Books and courses are available for the following specialties:

MRCP Part 1 and Part 2, MRCPCH Part 1 and Part 2, MRCS, MRCOG, MRCGP, DRCOG, MRCPsych, DCH, FRCA and PLAB.

For further details contact:

PasTest, Freepost, Knutsford, Cheshire WA16 7BR
Tel: 01565 752000   Fax: 01565 650264
E-mail: enquiries@pastest.co.uk
Web site: www.pastest.co.uk

Typeset by Breeze Limited, Manchester
Printed and bound by MPG Books Ltd, Bodmin Cornwall

CONTENTS

INTRODUCTION

PasTest's MRCP Part 1 Pocket Books are designed to help the busy examination candidate to make the most of every opportunity to revise. With this little book in your pocket, it is the work of a moment to open it, choose a question, decide upon your answers and then check the answer. Revising 'on the run' in this manner is both reassuring (if your answer is correct) and stimulating (if you find any gaps in your knowledge).

The MRCP Part 1 examination consists of two papers, each lasting three hours. Both papers contain 100 'Best of Five' questions (one answer is chosen from five options). Questions in each specialty are randomised across both papers. *No marks are deducted for a wrong answer.*

One-best answer/'Best of Five' MCQs
An important characteristic of one-best answer MCQs is that they can be designed to test application of knowledge and clinical problem-solving rather than just the recall of facts. This should change (for the better) the ways in which candidates prepare for MRCP Part 1.

Each one-best MCQ has a question stem, which usually contains clinical information, followed by five branches. All five branches are typically homologous (e.g. all diagnoses, all laboratory investigations, all antibiotics etc) and should be set out in a logical order (e.g. alphabetical). Candidates are asked to select the ONE branch that is the best answer to the question. A response is not required to the other four branches. The answer sheet is, therefore, slightly different to that used for true/false MCQs.

A good strategy that can be used with many well-written one-best MCQs is to try to reach the correct answer without first scrutinising the five options. If you can then find the answer you have reached in the option list, then you are probably correct.

One-best answer MCQs are quicker to answer than multiple true/false MCQs because only one response is needed for each question. Even though the question stem for one-best answer MCQs is usually longer than for true/false questions, and therefore takes a little longer to read carefully, it is reasonable to set more one-best than true/false MCQs for the same exam duration – in this instance 60 true/false and 100 one-best are used in exams of 2 hours.

Application of Knowledge and Clinical Problem-Solving
Unlike true/false MCQs, which test mainly the recall of knowledge, one-best answer questions test application and problem-solving. This makes them more effective test items and is one of the reasons why testing time can be reduced. In order to answer

these questions correctly, it is necessary to apply basic knowledge – not just be able to remember it. Furthermore, candidates who cannot reach the correct answer by applying their knowledge are much less likely to be able to choose the right answer by guessing than they were with true/false MCQs. This gives a big advantage to the best candidates, who have good knowledge and can apply it in clinical situations.

Books like the ones in this series, which consist of 'Best of Five' in subject categories, can help you to focus on specific topics and to isolate your weaknesses. You should plan a revision timetable to help you spread your time evenly over the range of subjects likely to appear in the examination. PasTest's *Essential Revision Notes for MRCP* by P Kalra will provide you with essential notes on all aspects of the syllabus.

CONTRIBUTORS

SECOND EDITION

Basic Sciences
Shani Esmail BSc MB Chir MRCP, Clinical Research Fellow in Clinical Pharmacology and Therapeutics, Western General Hospital, Edinburgh
David W Ray PhD MRCP, Senior Lecturer in Medicine And Honorary Consultant in Endocrinology University of Manchester and Manchester Royal Infirmary, Manchester
Edward Tobias BSc MBChB MRCP PhD, Glaxo-Wellcome Clinical Research Fellow And Honorary Consultant in Medical Genetics Department of Medical Genetics University of Glasgow. Glasgow

Neurology
Geraint Rees MRCP PhD, Wellcome Senior Clinical Fellow, Institute of Cognitive Neuroscience, University of London, London

Psychiatry
M Zoha MB ChB MRCPsych, Consultant Psychiatrist, St Charles Hospital, London

FIRST EDITION

Basic Sciences
David W Ray PhD MRCP, Senior Lecturer in Medicine And Honorary Consultant in Endocrinology University of Manchester and Manchester Royal Infirmary, Manchester
Edward Tobias BSc MBChB MRCP PhD, Glaxo-Wellcome Clinical Research Fellow And Honorary Consultant in Medical Genetics Department of Medical Genetics University of Glasgow, Glasgow
Donal O Donoghue Consultant Renal Physician, Department of Renal Medicine, Hope Hospital, Salford

Neurology
Geraint Rees MRCP PhD, Wellcome Senior Clinical Fellow, Institute of Cognitive Neuroscience, University of London, London
Christopher Moore MRCP, MRC Training Fellow and Honorary Senior Registrar, Manchester Royal Infirmary, Manchester

Psychiatry
M Zoha MB ChB MRCPsych, Consultant Psychiatrist, St Charles Hospital, London
Richard S Hopkins MRCPsych, Lecturer in Psychiatry and Honorary Senior Registrar, Withington Hospital, Manchester

BASIC SCIENCES

Best of Five

Questions

BASIC SCIENCES: 'BEST OF FIVE' QUESTIONS

For each of the questions select the ONE most appropriate answer from the options provided.

1.1 **A 39-year-old man is referred to the Neurology Department with a history of chorea, ataxia and cognitive decline. He is subsequently diagnosed with Huntington's disease. Which one of the following statements regarding this disorder is correct?**

- [ ] A   It is autosomal recessively inherited
- [ ] B   All daughters of affected men are affected but none of their sons
- [ ] C   All his offspring have a 50% chance of inheriting the disease
- [ ] D   There is no male-to-male transmission
- [ ] E   It is caused by a mitochondrial DNA mutation

1.2 **A 17-year-old boy presents with a history of learning difficulties, behavioural problems, dysarthria and arthropathy. On examination, he has a marked tremor and Kayser–Fleischer corneal rings. He is investigated, and a diagnosis of Wilson's disease is made. Which one of the following statements regarding this disorder is correct?**

- [ ] A   The gene is located on chromosome 6
- [ ] B   If an affected individual marries an unaffected individual 50% of the children will be carriers
- [ ] C   Affected men can only have normal sons and carrier daughters
- [ ] D   Affected cases are usually males carrying the gene or (rarely) homozygous females
- [ ] E   When both parents carry the gene each of their offspring has a 1 in 4 (25%) chance of being affected and a 50% chance of being a carrier

1.3 A 29-year-old woman is admitted to the Emergency Department with a history of headache, photophobia, drowsiness and seizures. On examination she is pyrexial and confused. She has photophobia and neck stiffness. CT head scan suggests some temporal lobe swelling is present. No haemorrhage, infarct or mass lesion is seen. You perform a lumbar puncture and send off her CSF for MC&S, Gram stain, protein, glucose and virology. You are concerned she may have meningoencephalitis, and ask the labs to do herpes simplex virus (HSV) PCR. You start her on intravenous aciclovir, ceftriaxone and benzylpenicillin and admit her to the Intensive Care Unit (ITU). Which one of the following statements regarding the polymerase chain reaction (PCR) is correct?

☐ A   It occurs at 40 °C

☐ B   It uses heat-labile DNA polymerase derived from *Thermus aquaticus*

☐ C   It can be used to amplify RNA directly

☐ D   It allows specific DNA sequences to be amplified from a single cell

☐ E   It involves cleavage of DNA with restriction enzymes, gel electrophoresis then visualisation on an autoradiograph following hybridisation with a specific DNA or RNA probe

1.4 A 56-year-old lady is referred to the Cardiology Clinic with a history of exertional chest pain. She undergoes an exercise ECG during which she exercises for 2 minutes and 14 seconds. The test is terminated because of chest pain and ST depression in the anterolateral leads. She is referred for coronary angiography. Which one of the following regarding the coronary circulation is correct?

☐ A   The right coronary artery arises from the posterior aortic cusp

☐ B   The left coronary artery usually arises from the anterior aortic sinus

☐ C   The left coronary artery usually bifurcates into the left anterior descending (LAD) artery and the circumflex artery

☐ D   The left coronary artery usually supplies the atrioventricular (AV) node

☐ E   The left anterior descending artery (LAD) gives off a posterior descending branch

1.5 **A 22-year-old woman is admitted to the Emergency Department following a paracetamol overdose. She has also slashed her left wrist, severing the median nerve. Which one of the following signs would be consistent with this injury?**

- ☐ A Wasting and paralysis of the hypothenar muscles of the left hand
- ☐ B Loss of sensation over the palmar aspect of the left little finger
- ☐ C Paralysis of the intrinsic hand muscles (apart from the lateral two lumbricals) on the left
- ☐ D Wrist drop
- ☐ E Paralysis of the thenar muscles, ie opponens pollicis, abductor pollicis brevis and flexor pollicis brevis

1.6 **A 55-year-old man is a patient on the Neurology Ward. He has noticed some deterioration in his vision lately. On examination of his visual fields he has a left homonymous superior quadrantanopia. Which one of the following is the most likely cause?**

- ☐ A Pituitary tumour compressing the optic chiasma
- ☐ B A lesion in the right parietal lobe
- ☐ C Thrombotic stroke affecting the posterior cerebral artery distribution
- ☐ D Temporal lobe lesion
- ☐ E Optic neuritis

1.7 **A female patient presents with galactorrhoea. Which one of the following medications would be most likely to cause this?**

- ☐ A Tamoxifen
- ☐ B Co-careldopa
- ☐ C Cyclizine
- ☐ D Bromocriptine
- ☐ E Metoclopramide

1.8 You review a 55-year-old man in the Cardiology Clinic. At his last hospital admission he was commenced on digoxin therapy. Which of the following statements concerning this drug are correct?

☐ A   It acts predominantly at the sinus node

☐ B   It has been shown to reduce mortality in patients with heart failure

☐ C   It is contraindicated in Wolff–Parkinson–White syndrome

☐ D   'Reversed tick' ST-segment depression on the ECG is pathognomonic of digoxin toxicity

☐ E   It will cardiovert atrial fibrillation

1.9 A 65-year-old man who has been attending the Cardiology Clinic presents with increasing shortness of breath on exertion, a reduced appetite and skin discoloration. His investigations are as follows: haemoglobin 13 g/dl, WCC 7 × 10⁹/l, platelets 190 × 10⁹/l, sodium 135 mmol/l, potassium 4.1 mmol/l, urea 8.0 mmol/l, creatinine 100 μmol/l, AST 160 U/l, ALP 180 U/l, albumin 39 g/l, bilirubin 48 μmol/l, FT4 24 pmol/l, TSH 0.2 mU/l.

Pulmonary function tests (PFTs):

	Actual	Predicted
FEV$_1$	2.8 l	4.0 l
FVC	3.1 l	5.0 l
FEV$_1$/FVC ratio – 90%		
T$_{LCO}$	0.7	1.6

Echocardiography shows an enlarged left atrium and a normal-sized left ventricle with good function and normal valves. Which of the following provides the best explanation for this patient's presentation?

☐ A   Congestive cardiac failure (CCF)

☐ B   Chest infection

☐ C   Hyperthyroidism

☐ D   Hereditary haemochromatosis

☐ E   Amiodarone toxicity

1.10 Which one of the following would be most likely to lead to these results: sodium 137 mmol/l, potassium 5.0 mmol/l, urea 5.2 mmol/l, creatinine 95 μmol/l, glucose 1.9 mmol/l?

☐ A   Polycystic ovarian syndrome

☐ B   Haemochromatosis

☐ C   Prednisolone treatment

☐ D   Metformin treatment

☐ E   Pituitary insufficiency

1.11 A 42-year-old publican is on holiday in southern Spain. Shortly after arrival he develops a blistering rash on his face. He had a similar rash last summer. His investigations are as follows: Hb 12.0 g/dl, WCC 8.0×10^9/l, platelets 82×10^9/l, albumin 30 g/l, bilirubin 15 μmol/l, AST 30 U/l, ALP 100 U/l, GGT 85 U/l. Which one of the following is the most likely diagnosis?

☐ A   Fixed drug eruption

☐ B   Sunburn

☐ C   Chronic alcoholic liver disease

☐ D   Systemic lupus erythematosus

☐ E   Porphyria cutanea tarda

1.12 A 22-year-old woman is admitted to the Emergency Department. Her plasma biochemistry is as follows: sodium 138 mmol/l, potassium 4.0 mmol/l, urea 5.0 mmol/l, creatinine 100 μmol/l, bicarbonate 18 mmol/l, chloride 105 mmol/l, glucose 5.0 mmol/l, plasma osmolality 307 mosmol/kg. Which one of the following is most likely to have caused these results?

☐ A   Type 2 renal tubular acidosis (RTA)

☐ B   Addison's disease

☐ C   Aspirin overdose

☐ D   Conn's syndrome

☐ E   Ethanol toxicity

1.13 Which one of the listed conditions would be most likely to produce the following arterial blood gas results: pH 7.49, Pao_2 12.3 kPa, $Paco_2$ 5.5 kPa, bicarbonate 34 mmol/l?

☐ A   Renal failure

☐ B   Anxiety attack

☐ C   Addison's disease

☐ D   Conn's syndrome

☐ E   Salicylate poisoning

1.14 A 36-year-old man is referred to the Rheumatology Clinic with a ten-year history of worsening lower back pain. Over the last year he has noticed pain in both knees. He also complains that his sweat is dark and stains his clothing. He has no history of rashes, alopecia, mouth or genital ulcers or diarrhoea. He did not complain of any eye problems. He had dysuria after a trip to Amsterdam at the age of 20 but this cleared up after treatment with oxytetracycline. He had no other PMH of note. On examination, abnormal pigmentation of his ears and sclerae is noted. He has lost his lumbar lordosis and lumbar spine flexion is reduced. His knee joints are swollen, with bilateral effusions. Examination of the rest of the musculoskeletal system is normal, as are cardiovascular, respiratory, gastrointestinal and neurological examinations. His investigations show the following: haemoglobin 13.5 g/dl, WCC 5×10^9/l, platelets 200×10^9/l, ESR 30 mm/hour, corrected calcium 2.3 mmol/l, phosphate 0.8 mmol/l, alkaline phosphatase 90 U/l, albumin 40 g/l, glucose 3.8 mmol/l. X-rays reveal loss of lumbar lordosis and intervertebral disc calcification. Urinalysis shows glucose ++, no protein. Which one of the following is the most likely diagnosis?

☐ A   Ankylosing spondylitis

☐ B   Alkaptonuria (ochronosis)

☐ C   Haemochromatosis

☐ D   Osteoarthritis

☐ E   Reiter's syndrome

1.15 **Which one of the following would be consistent with these results: sodium 137 mmol/l, potassium 3.4 mmol/l, urea 7.0 mmol/l, creatinine 106 μmol/l, chloride 107 mmol/l, bicarbonate 18 mmol/l?**

☐ A   Diabetic ketoacidosis

☐ B   Severe diarrhoea

☐ C   Alcoholic ketoacidosis

☐ D   Salicylate poisoning

☐ E   Lactic acidosis

1.16 **A 30-year-old lady presents with left loin pain. Her only other history is that of two vertebral crush fractures. Her investigations are: urinalysis blood +++, pH 7, serum sodium 135 mmol/l, potassium 2.8 mmol/l, urea 5.7 mmol/l, creatinine 107 μmol/l, chloride 115 mmol/l, bicarbonate 9 mmol/l. What is the most likely underlying diagnosis?**

☐ A   Renal calculus

☐ B   Diabetic ketoacidosis (DKA)

☐ C   Type 1 (distal) renal tube acidosis (RTA)

☐ D   Urinary tract infection (UTI)

☐ E   Type 2 (proximal) RTA

1.17 **A 28-year-old woman is admitted to the Emergency Department following a seizure. She has had crampy abdominal pain and vomiting for the last two days. Previously she has been hospitalised for depression. She last went to her GP five days ago, when she was prescribed a new oral contraceptive. Her blood tests show: haemoglobin 12.1 g/dl, WCC 12.5 × 10^9/l, platelets 370 × 10^9/l, sodium 129 mmol/l, potassium 4.1 mmol/l, urea 6.6 mmol/l, creatinine 100 μmol/l. Which one of the following is the most likely underlying diagnosis?**

☐ A   Drug-induced convulsions

☐ B   Encephalitis

☐ C   Urinary tract infection

☐ D   Acute intermittent porphyria

☐ E   Hyponatraemia

1.18   **You review a male patient with recently diagnosed liver cirrhosis. A liver screen has been done, which suggests chronic hepatitis C infection. Which one of the following statements regarding hepatitis C liver disease is true?**

☐   A   Hepatitis C is a DNA virus

☐   B   Chronic liver disease occurs in 50–80% of those infected

☐   C   Interferon-α results in clearance of the virus in 90% of patients

☐   D   Fulminant hepatitis is common

☐   E   Transmission is usually faecal–oral

1.19   **A 52-year-old man is referred to the Neurology Clinic with a history of rapid memory loss and decline in cognitive function, myoclonus and ataxia. He is assessed and investigated, and a diagnosis of sporadic Creutzfeldt–Jakob disease is made. Which one of the following statements regarding this disease and its cause is correct?**

☐   A   It is caused by a virus

☐   B   The causative agent is denatured by heat, ionising radiation and formaldehyde

☐   C   It characteristically has a slow, indolent course

☐   D   Most cases may be diagnosed by CT scanning

☐   E   It may be transmitted by corneal grafts

1.20   **A 32-year-old man has hepatitis B. Which one of the following statements is true of this disease?**

☐   A   The virus only infects hepatocytes

☐   B   80% of those infected develop chronic hepatitis B infection

☐   C   IgG HbcAb indicates previous infection, now cleared

☐   D   Blood levels of HbeAg correlate with infectivity

☐   E   Patients who are immunodeficient are more likely to develop fulminant hepatic failure than those who are immunocompetent

1.21   You have joined Médecins Sans Frontières and have been posted to tropical Africa. One of your patients, a 19-year-old woman, presents with a sore throat, malaise and anorexia. On examination she has a low-grade fever, cervical lymphadenopathy and a bluish-white membrane covering her pharynx. Eleven days later her voice assumes a nasal quality and fluid regurgitates through her nose. Which one of the following statements regarding her diagnosis is correct?

☐ A   The causative organism is an invasive aerobic Gram-negative rod

☐ B   She is likely to have polio

☐ C   Treatment should only be started when there is laboratory confirmation of the diagnosis

☐ D   Treatment with antitoxin is unhelpful

☐ E   Severe complications occur due to the production of an exotoxin that inhibits protein synthesis

1.22   A 50-year-old man is admitted to the Emergency Department. His arterial blood gases are: pH 7.23, PaO_2 7.0 kPa, $PaCO_2$ 8.1 kPa. Which one of the following would be most likely to produce these results?

☐ A   Pulmonary haemorrhage

☐ B   Pulmonary embolism

☐ C   Pneumothorax

☐ D   An overdose of diazepam

☐ E   Asthma

1.23   Which one of the following displaces the oxygen-haemoglobin dissociation curve to the left?

☐ A   An increase in the pH

☐ B   A rise in the temperature

☐ C   Increased lactate production

☐ D   A rise in $PaCO_2$

☐ E   Chronic hypoxia due to cyanotic heart disease

1.24 You review a 65-year-old man with type 2 diabetes in the clinic. His diabetes is not controlled on maximal oral hypoglycaemic therapy, and you would like to start him on insulin. Which one of the following is a metabolic effect of insulin?

- ☐ A   Increased lipolysis in adipose tissue
- ☐ B   Increased ketogenesis in the liver
- ☐ C   Decreased glycogen synthesis in liver and muscle
- ☐ D   Increased protein synthesis
- ☐ E   Decreased glucose uptake into tissues

1.25 You are involved in running a hypertension screening programme in your local area. Two thousand people, aged 30–80, are screened. Both the mean and the median of the systolic blood pressure distribution are approximately 145 mmHg and the standard deviation is 22 mmHg. Which one of the following statements is correct?

- ☐ A   5% of the subjects will have a systolic blood pressure greater than 189 mmHg
- ☐ B   Approximately 95% of the subjects have systolic blood pressures between 101 and 189 mmHg
- ☐ C   Approximately 68% of the subjects have systolic blood pressures between 101 and 189 mmHg
- ☐ D   99% of the observations lie within 2.6 standard errors of the mean
- ☐ E   The distribution is assymetric

1.26 A new oral hypoglycaemic is administered to patients with type 2 diabetes in a clinical trial. Which one of the following statements is correct?

- ☐ A   A fall in plasma glucose with a probability value of $P > 0.05$ would indicate that the drug has a significant effect
- ☐ B   Parametric tests should be used on data that has a skewed distribution
- ☐ C   The statistical significance of the fall in blood glucose may be analysed by a paired Student's t-test
- ☐ D   If the P value = 0.01, 1 in 20 studies would be expected to show a significant effect of the drug on blood glucose by chance alone
- ☐ E   In a single-blind study neither the researcher nor the patient knows which treatment the patient has been randomised to

1.27 **The table below shows the results from a screening test for bowel cancer:**

Screening test result	True Diagnosis		
	Bowel cancer	No bowel cancer	Total
Positive	50	11	61
Negative	2	4939	4941
Total	52	4950	5002

Which one of the following statements regarding this screening test are correct?

- ☐ A   The sensitivity of the screening test is 82%
- ☐ B   The sensitivity of the screening test is 96%
- ☐ C   The positive predictive value is 96%
- ☐ D   The negative predictive value is 82%
- ☐ E   The sensitivity and specificity of the screening test depend on the disease prevalence

1.28 **Hormones are capable of acting at distant sites via specific, high-affinity receptors. Concerning hormone action, which one of the following statements is true?**

- ☐ A   ACTH receptors are coupled to G proteins
- ☐ B   Cortisol binds to the mineralocorticoid receptor
- ☐ C   Insulin acts by causing dimerisation of two subunits of the insulin receptor, and stimulating adenylate cyclase
- ☐ D   PAR alpha binds to the thiazolidine group of drugs
- ☐ E   Thyroid hormone binds to a membrane receptor

1.29 **In thyrotoxicosis, appropriate management depends on the aetiology, and associated pathologies. Which of the following statements is true?**

- ☐ A   Carbimazole is contraindicated in pregnancy
- ☐ B   Graves' disease is associated with myasthenia gravis
- ☐ C   Graves' ophthalmopathy requires high-dose steroid treatment
- ☐ D   Radioactive iodine improves exophthalmos in Graves' disease
- ☐ E   Toxic multinodular goitre may go into long-term remission following a course of carbimazole

1.30 **The clinical diagnosis of adrenal insufficiency is suggested by which one of the following?**

☐ A   Hypertension

☐ B   Hypoglycaemia

☐ C   Hypokalaemia

☐ D   Neutrophilia

☐ E   Pallor

1.31 **In the clinical evaluation of gynaecomastia which one of the following underlying diagnoses is unlikely?**

☐ A   Amiodarone

☐ B   Klinefelter's syndrome

☐ C   Renal failure

☐ D   Spironolactone

☐ E   Testicular malignancy

1.32 **In the management of acromegaly which one of the following statements is correct?**

☐ A   90% of patients respond to long-acting somatostatin analogue treatment

☐ B   Diabetes mellitus occurs in < 5% of patients

☐ C   Hypercholesterolaemia is common

☐ D   Patients with pituitary microadenomas can be cured in 50% of cases

☐ E   Suprasellar extension prevents a trans-sphenoidal surgical approach

1.33 **Concerning monoclonal antibodies which one of the following statements is not true?**

☐ A   They are used to limit transplant rejection

☐ B   They are made using human B lymphocytes

☐ C   They can be used to activate T lymphocytes *in vitro*

☐ D   They can be used to detect proteins in histological sections

☐ E   They can be used to measure hormones in blood

1.34 **Which one of the following is a characteristic of mitochondrial diseases?**

☐ A They cause hypothyroidism

☐ B They cause ketoacidosis

☐ C They cause 'ragged red' fibres in skeletal muscle

☐ D They involve the renal tubule

☐ E They are paternally inherited

1.35 **Concerning genetic anticipation:**

☐ A It is characteristic of neurofibromatosis type 1

☐ B It is not seen with fragile X syndrome

☐ C It refers to earlier diagnosis due to improved awareness

☐ D It occurs in Turner's syndrome

☐ E It results from amplification of triplet repeats within genes

1.36 **Concerning the regulation of gene expression, which one of the following statements is correct?**

☐ A Introns are not transcribed into mRNA

☐ B Mammalian mRNA tends to be polycistronic

☐ C Mutations in the DNA sequence encoding a gene always result in changes in the amino acid sequence of the resulting protein

☐ D RNA polymerase II gives rise to protein encoding mRNA

☐ E The majority of cellular RNA is mRNA

1.37 **Tumour necrosis factor-α:**

☐ A Activates the nuclear factor kappa B (NFkB) transcription factor

☐ B Binds a single, specific receptor

☐ C Inhibits expression of interleukin-1 (IL-1)

☐ D Is useful treatment for rheumatoid arthritis

☐ E Leads to enhanced insulin sensitivity

1.38   In rheumatoid arthritis, which one of the following is true?

☐ A   Association of seropositivity with HLA-DR1

☐ B   Concordance rate of > 60% for identical twins

☐ C   Peak incidence in the third decade

☐ D   Progression from predominantly small peripheral joint disease to involve more proximal, larger joints

☐ E   Sacroiliac joint disease is common

1.39   In polymyalgia rheumatica:

☐ A   Electromyography (EMG) studies detect a typical abnormality

☐ B   Night sweats and fever make the diagnosis unlikely

☐ C   Half of patients are aged less than 60 years

☐ D   Patients have a characteristic reduction in circulating CD8+ T lymphocytes

☐ E   The response to prednisolone is helpful in diagnosis

1.40   The HLA-B27 molecule is:

☐ A   A class II major histocompatibility antigen

☐ B   Expressed on antigen-presenting dendritic cells

☐ C   Found in 50% of Caucasians with ankylosing spondylitis

☐ D   Over-represented in Crohn's disease

☐ E   Over-represented in Whipple's disease

1.41   Vasculitis may be caused by different disease processes. Which one of the following statements is not true?

☐ A   Antibodies to proteinase-3 are specific for vasculitis

☐ B   Churg–Strauss syndrome patients typically present with asthma

☐ C   Polyarteritis nodosa mainly affects small vessels

☐ D   There is a seasonal peak in incidence in North America

☐ E   Wegener's granulomatosis affects the small vessels of the kidney

1.42 **Systemic lupus erythematosus (SLE) is a systemic inflammatory disease. Which one of the following statements is true concerning SLE?**

- ☐ A 15% have Raynaud's phenomenon
- ☐ B C-reactive protein is a useful marker of disease activity
- ☐ C It is less common in Klinefelter's syndrome
- ☐ D High frequencies of disease are seen in women of Chinese ancestry
- ☐ E The skin is affected in < 50% of cases

1.43 **Concerning urinary sediment, which one of the following is correct?**

- ☐ A < 100 white cells per ml is normal
- ☐ B Cystine crystals are often found in normal urine
- ☐ C Hyaline casts consist of Tamm–Horsfall protein
- ☐ D Oxalate crystals in the urine suggest renal disease
- ☐ E Red cells always indicate renal tract disease

1.44 **Patients with renal failure may require drug treatment in addition to haemodialysis. Which one of the following drugs is dialysed by haemodialysis?**

- ☐ A Aciclovir
- ☐ B Erythromycin
- ☐ C Propranolol
- ☐ D Vancomycin
- ☐ E Warfarin

1.45 **In the evaluation of a patient with raised urea and creatinine, pre-renal failure is unlikely if there is:**

- ☐ A Decreased pulmonary wedge pressure
- ☐ B Postural hypotension
- ☐ C Urine osmolality > 500 mosm/l
- ☐ D Urine sodium > 20 mmol/l
- ☐ E Urine to plasma urea ratio of > 8

1.46 **Concerning adult polycystic kidney disease, which one of the following is true?**

☐ A 10% of affected patients will also have hepatic cysts

☐ B Abdominal pain is a common presenting feature

☐ C It has autosomal recessive inheritance

☐ D Generally results in end-stage renal failure in the third decade

☐ E Spontaneous haematuria is unusual

1.47 **Concerning acid-base function of the kidney, which one of the following statements is not true?**

☐ A > 80% of all filtered bicarbonate ions are actively recovered

☐ B In distal renal tubular acidosis (RTA type 1) there is normal anion gap, metabolic acidosis and urinary pH > 5.5

☐ C Nephrocalcinosis suggests type 1 or distal RTA

☐ D Proximal renal tubular acidosis is usually an inherited condition

☐ E The proximal nephron actively secretes hydrogen ions, in contrast to the distal nephron

1.48 **With regard to human immunodeficiency virus (HIV):**

☐ A CD8 cells become depleted as disease progresses

☐ B HIV-1 and HIV-2 are closely related, and cause similar disease progression

☐ C HIV gains entry to the cell via the TNF receptor

☐ D It is a lentivirus

☐ E The HIV genome contains circular DNA

1.49 **Concerning pneumococcal disease:**

☐ A Pneumococcal meningitis is associated with similar mortality rates to meningococcal meningitis in industrialised countries

☐ B Pneumococcal otitis media is usually associated with neutrophil leucocytosis

☐ C Pneumococcal pneumonia shows no seasonal variation in temperate countries

☐ D *Pneumococcus* is a Gram-negative organism

☐ E Sickle cell disease predisposes to pneumococcal infection, and antibiotic prophylaxis is ineffective

1.50 **Concerning herpes simplex virus infection, which one of the following is correct?**

☐ A 10% of herpes encephalitis cases are due to reactivation of virus

☐ B Antibody titres are helpful in making management decisions

☐ C It is caused by a single-stranded DNA virus

☐ D Herpes meningitis is a relatively benign condition in adults

☐ E Precedes 50% of all cases of erythema multiforme

1.51 **Concerning meningococcal disease, which one of the following statements is untrue?**

☐ A Haemorrhagic skin lesions are a late feature of septicaemia

☐ B Identification of Gram-positive diplococci on lumbar puncture suggests meningococcal meningitis

☐ C Meningococcaemia is associated with neutrophilia

☐ D Rifampicin eradicates nasal carriage in fewer than 30% of contacts

☐ E Transmission is usually by respiratory droplet

1.52 **Fever in a patient returning from foreign travel is unlikely to be due to typhoid fever if which one of the following clinical features is present?**

☐ A Altered mental state

☐ B Associated headache

☐ C Change in bowel habit

☐ D Haematuria

☐ E Lack of diurnal variation in the temperature

1.53 **Which one of the following is true of Marfan's syndrome?**

☐ A Aortic dissection is a recognised complication

☐ B Mutations in the collagen gene are typical

☐ C New mutations in the gene are rare

☐ D The inheritance pattern is X-linked dominant

☐ E The mutations generally occur at the same position within the gene

1.54 **Blood vessel rupture is not a recognised complication of which one of the following genetic conditions?**

- ☐ A   Ehlers–Danlos syndrome
- ☐ B   Marfan's syndrome
- ☐ C   Polycystic kidney disease
- ☐ D   Pseudoxanthoma elasticum
- ☐ E   Velocardiofacial syndrome

1.55 **In Klinefelter's syndrome, which one of the following is correct?**

- ☐ A   Severe learning difficulties are common
- ☐ B   Significant gynaecomastia is present in almost all cases
- ☐ C   The incidence is about 1 in 50 000 newborn males
- ☐ D   There is a 10–15% chance of recurrence of a chromosomal abnormality after the birth of a child with Klinefelter's syndrome
- ☐ E   There is no increase in the incidence of homosexuality

1.56 **Which one of the following conditions is correctly paired with the gene responsible for that condition?**

- ☐ A   Achondroplasia   *SMN* (survival motor neurone)
- ☐ B   Congenital muscular dystrophy   sarcoglycans gene
- ☐ C   HNPCC   *hMLH1*
- ☐ D   Limb-girdle muscular dystrophy   merosin gene
- ☐ E   Spinal muscular atrophy   *FGFR3*

1.57 **Which one of the following is true of nuclear DNA?**

- ☐ A   Approximately 97% codes for proteins
- ☐ B   Base-pairing is mediated by covalent bonds
- ☐ C   Coding sequences are interrupted by non-coding exons
- ☐ D   It exists predominantly as a nucleoprotein complex
- ☐ E   Sugar and phosphate molecules are linked together by hydrogen bonds

NEUROLOGY

Best of Five

Questions

NEUROLOGY: 'BEST OF FIVE' QUESTIONS

For each of the questions select the ONE most appropriate answer from the options provided.

2.1   An obese 45-year-old woman presents with headaches and visual loss, and is found to have papilloedema. A CT head scan is normal. What is the most likely diagnosis?

☐ A   Optic neuritis

☐ B   Benign intracranial hypertension

☐ C   Migraine

☐ D   Normal-pressure hydrocephalus

☐ E   Acromegaly

2.2   A 56-year-old man presents with altered sensation in the right little finger and lateral aspect of the palm. There is weakness of the small muscles of the hand. Which nerve is most likely to be damaged?

☐ A   Median nerve

☐ B   Anterior interosseous nerve

☐ C   Radial nerve

☐ D   Ulnar nerve

☐ E   Axillary nerve

2.3   A 22-year-old woman has a two-day history of frontal headache and blurring of vision in the right eye, aggravated by eye movement. Her visual acuities are 6/18 (right) and 6/5 (left) with a right afferent pupillary defect. What is the most likely appearance of the optic disc in the right eye?

☐ A   Haemorrhagic

☐ B   Large cup

☐ C   Swollen

☐ D   Pale

☐ E   Normal

2.4 **A 33-year-old man presents with a sudden-onset, severe occipital headache; there are no abnormal clinical signs and CT (head) is normal. What is the most important investigation to perform urgently?**

- ☐ A Magnetic resonance imaging (MRI) of the brain
- ☐ B Electroencephalogram (EEG)
- ☐ C Lumbar puncture
- ☐ D Serum creatine kinase estimation
- ☐ E ECG

2.5 **A 58-year-old man presents with progressive memory loss over two years, occasional incontinence of urine and a shuffling gait. What is a CT scan of the brain most likely to show?**

- ☐ A Multiple white matter lesions
- ☐ B Parasagittal meningioma
- ☐ C Temporal lobe glioma
- ☐ D Communicating hydrocephalus
- ☐ E Normal appearance

2.6 **A 63-year-old man is found to have a left homonymous hemianopia. What structure is likely to be damaged?**

- ☐ A Left occipital lobe
- ☐ B Right occipital lobe
- ☐ C Left lateral geniculate nucleus
- ☐ D Optic chiasm
- ☐ E Left optic nerve

2.7 **A 23-year-old man presents with the rapid onset of right leg weakness. There is decreased proprioception in the right leg and absent sensation to pinprick in the left leg. What is the most likely diagnosis?**

- ☐ A Guillain–Barré syndrome
- ☐ B Intramedullary spinal cord glioma
- ☐ C Brown-Séquard syndrome
- ☐ D Anterior spinal artery occlusion
- ☐ E Lumbosacral disc herniation

2.8 A 56-year-old diabetic presents with horizontal diplopia, worse on looking to the right. The outer image disappears when the right eye is covered. Which nerve is most likely to have been affected?

☐ A   Right oculomotor

☐ B   Left abducens

☐ C   Right abducens

☐ D   Left trochlear

☐ E   Right trochlear

2.9 A new diagnostic test for variant Creutzfeldt–Jakob disease (vCJD) has recently been published. What term describes the proportion of patients with confirmed variant CJD that will be identified by the test?

☐ A   Accuracy

☐ B   Negative predictive value

☐ C   Positive predictive value

☐ D   Sensitivity

☐ E   Specificity

2.10 A 67-year-old woman has repeated stabbing pain in the right cheek, precipitated by chewing or washing her face. What is the best initial treatment for her condition?

☐ A   Carbamazepine

☐ B   Propranolol

☐ C   Benzhexol

☐ D   Botulinum toxin

☐ E   Methotrexate

2.11 A 67-year-old man presents with sudden onset of unsteadiness, dizziness and weakness. He has a right Horner's syndrome, right-sided pyramidal weakness, and loss of pinprick sensation on his left side. What is the most likely diagnosis?

☐ A   Posterior communicating artery aneurysm

☐ B   Occipital haemorrhage

☐ C   Posterior inferior cerebellar artery occlusion

☐ D   Pontine haemorrhage

☐ E   Carotid arterial dissection

2.12 A 23-year-old man has been having continuous grand mal seizures for 15 minutes, having been given lorazepam 4mg intravenously five minutes ago. What is the most appropriate immediate treatment?

- ☐ A Intravenous diazepam 10 mg
- ☐ B Intravenous lorazepam 2 mg
- ☐ C Intravenous phenytoin 15 mg/kg
- ☐ D Oral phenytoin 300 mg
- ☐ E Intravenous phenobarbital (phenobarbitone) 1 mg/kg

2.13 A 58-year-old right-handed woman has finger agnosia, left-right disorientation, acalculia and agraphia. Which cortical structure is most likely to be damaged?

- ☐ A Left angular gyrus
- ☐ B Anterior cingulate gyrus
- ☐ C Right angular gyrus
- ☐ D Left fusiform gyrus
- ☐ E Right fusiform gyrus

2.14 A 58-year-old man has memory loss that has progressed rapidly over three months. He is profoundly ataxic. What is the most likely diagnosis?

- ☐ A Pick's disease
- ☐ B Creutzfeldt–Jakob disease
- ☐ C Lewy body dementia
- ☐ D Wilson's disease
- ☐ E Corticobasal dementia

2.15 A 23-year-old woman suffers a single unprovoked seizure. What advice is most appropriate to give her regarding driving a private motor vehicle?

- ☐ A No driving only if there is a further seizure
- ☐ B No driving only if a structural lesion is confirmed
- ☐ C No driving only if there are EEG abnormalities
- ☐ D No driving for three years
- ☐ E No driving for one year

2.16 A 38-year-old man with migraine takes sumatriptan but is finding that the frequency of his migraines has increased recently to six to eight per month. What is the most appropriate medication to consider adding?

☐ A   Haloperidol

☐ B   Rizatriptan

☐ C   Aspirin

☐ D   Carbamazepine

☐ E   Propranolol

2.17 A 23-year-old man develops foot drop and disturbance of sensation over the dorsum of the foot. What nerve in the lower limb is most likely to have been damaged?

☐ A   Common peroneal

☐ B   Sciatic

☐ C   Tibial

☐ D   Obturator

☐ E   Femoral

2.18 A 54-year-old woman with ovarian carcinoma develops profound ataxia. MRI (brain) is normal. What blood test is most likely to aid in making a diagnosis?

☐ A   Anti-Hu antibodies

☐ B   Anti-Ro antibodies

☐ C   Anti-Yo antibodies

☐ D   Acetylcholine receptor antibodies

☐ E   Calcium channel antibodies

2.19 A 32-year-old man presents with a two-week history of gradually worsening vision in his right eye, associated with discomfort on left eye movements. Visual acuity is decreased in the right eye with a right afferent pupillary defect; fundi are normal. What is the most likely diagnosis?

☐ A   Orbital meningioma

☐ B   Pituitary tumour

☐ C   Tobacco amblyopia

☐ D   Optic neuritis

☐ E   Ischaemic optic neuropathy

2.20 A 37-year-old HIV-positive man complains of mild right-sided weakness for two weeks. CT (head) shows a hypodense lesion with ring enhancement in the left basal ganglia and frontal region. What is the most likely diagnosis?

- ☐ A Cerebral vasculitis
- ☐ B Neurocysticercosis
- ☐ C Toxoplasmosis
- ☐ D Neurosyphilis
- ☐ E Cytomegalovirus encephalitis

2.21 A 23-year-old woman presents with two episodes of non-sustained jerking of the left arm lasting a few minutes without loss of consciousness. MRI (brain) is normal. What is the most appropriate medication to commence?

- ☐ A Phenytoin
- ☐ B Levetiracetam
- ☐ C Carbamazepine
- ☐ D Lorazepam
- ☐ E Vigabatrin

2.22 A 48-year-old woman has recently taken antibiotics for sinusitis but develops vomiting and headache. CSF examination demonstrates 40 white cells (80% lymphocytes), protein 0.6 g/l (normal range 0.15–0.45 g/l), normal glucose and negative Gram stain. What is the most likely diagnosis?

- ☐ A Viral meningitis
- ☐ B Partially treated bacterial meningitis
- ☐ C Cryptococcal meningitis
- ☐ D Cerebral toxoplasmosis
- ☐ E Viral encephalitis

2.23 A 75-year-old man presents with an 18-month history of progressive difficulty using his right arm, slurred speech, difficulty walking and feeling dizzy on standing. He has a resting tremor of his right arm, dysarthria and mild postural hypotension. What is the most likely diagnosis?

☐ A   Shy–Drager syndrome

☐ B   Idiopathic Parkinson's disease

☐ C   Steele–Richardson–Olszewski syndrome

☐ D   Progressive supranuclear palsy

☐ E   Wilson's disease

2.24 A 54-year-old man presents with symptoms suggestive of myasthenia gravis, including fatiguable weakness in his upper limbs. Which of the following is the best investigation to confirm the diagnosis?

☐ A   Tensilon® test

☐ B   Muscle biopsy

☐ C   Visual-evoked potentials

☐ D   MRI of the brain

☐ E   Nerve conduction studies

2.25 A 43-year-old woman complains of unsteadiness, syncope, constipation and urinary retention. She was previously well, takes no medications and has no relevant family history. On physical examination you find bradykinesia, mild resting tremor, and severe postural hypotension. Which one of the following is the most likely diagnosis?

☐ A   Huntington's disease

☐ B   Idiopathic Parkinson's disease

☐ C   Multiple system atrophy

☐ D   Normal-pressure hydrocephalus

☐ E   Progressive supranuclear palsy

2.26   A 56-year-old man with poorly controlled diabetes complains of horizontal diplopia. You notice a subtle convergent strabismus. His diplopia is worse on looking to the right, and on covering his right eye he tells you that the outer image disappears. Which one of the following cranial nerves is the most likely site of the underlying lesion?

   ☐   A   Left abducens nerve

   ☐   B   Left oculomotor nerve

   ☐   C   Right abducens nerve

   ☐   D   Right oculomotor nerve

   ☐   E   Right trochlear nerve

2.27   A 58-year-old woman is brought to the Emergency Department unresponsive after collapsing at her home. Her husband reports that she felt well that morning, but developed a progressively severe headache. She has a history of hypertension and atrial fibrillation for which she is anticoagulated. On examination she has a blood pressure of 220/140 mmHg and has apnoea alternating with hyperpnoea. She responds only to noxious stimuli, with right-sided extensor posturing. She has papilloedema and an unreactive pupil on the left, diffuse hyper-reflexia and bilateral upgoing plantars. Which one of the following herniation syndromes is most consistent with her clinical presentation?

   ☐   A   Brainstem through the tentorial notch

   ☐   B   Cerebellar tonsils through the foramen magnum

   ☐   C   Cingulate gyrus beneath the falx

   ☐   D   Diencephalon through the tentorial notch

   ☐   E   Temporal lobe uncus across the tentorium

2.28   A 62-year-old man develops left-sided limb ataxia, left Horner's syndrome, nystagmus and loss of pain and temperature sensation on the right side of his face. Which artery is most likely to be occluded?

   ☐   A   Basilar artery

   ☐   B   Posterior cerebral artery

   ☐   C   Posterior inferior cerebellar artery

   ☐   D   Superior cerebellar artery

   ☐   E   Vertebral artery

2.29   A 31-year-old man gives a three-year history of increasing deafness and
        tinnitus in his right ear. He is a smoker and has no other medical history.
        On examination, his auditory acuity is grossly impaired on the left. Rinne's
        test shows air conduction to be greater than bone conduction. You notice
        no nystagmus, and balance is normal, but the left corneal reflex is absent.
        Which one of the following is the most likely diagnosis?

   ☐ A   Acoustic neuroma

   ☐ B   Basilar artery aneurysm

   ☐ C   Brainstem astrocytoma

   ☐ D   Multiple sclerosis

   ☐ E   Nasopharyngeal carcinoma

2.30   A 52-year-old woman presents with a three-month history of right-sided
        tingling, numbness and weakness. Her entire right side is completely numb,
        yet hypersensitive to touch. Five years earlier she underwent mastectomy
        for breast carcinoma. You find a hemiplegic gait, right hemianaesthesia to
        all sensory modalities, minimal weakness and flexor plantars. Which one of
        the following is most likely to be causing these symptoms and signs?

   ☐ A   Left posterior cerebral artery infarction

   ☐ B   Left postcentral gyrus metastasis

   ☐ C   Left thalamic metastasis

   ☐ D   Multiple sclerosis

   ☐ E   Right cerebellar infarction

2.31   A 26-year-old man, previously healthy, complains of progressive visual loss
        accompanied by intermittent central headaches. On examination you note
        a bitemporal inferior quadrantanopia, but no other neurological
        abnormalities. Which one of the following diagnoses is most likely?

   ☐ A   Craniopharyngioma

   ☐ B   Cushing's disease

   ☐ C   Optic neuritis

   ☐ D   Prolactinoma

   ☐ E   Retinitis pigmentosa

2.32   A 48-year-old hypertensive man tripped while playing football, and awoke the next day with severe foot drop. On examination, foot eversion is impaired and there is there is severe weakness of dorsiflexion. The ankle reflex is intact, and there is no evidence of sensory loss. Which one of the following structures is most likely to be damaged?

☐   A   Common peroneal nerve

☐   B   Femoral nerve

☐   C   L5/S1 nerve root

☐   D   Sciatic nerve

☐   E   Tibial nerve

2.33   A 36-year-old Asian man presents with a two-day history of sore throat, headache and vomiting. Two years previously he underwent splenectomy following a road traffic accident. On examination, he is confused, disoriented, febrile and photophobic. He is tachycardic and you notice a petechial rash on his upper arms, together with mild neck stiffness and a positive Kernig's sign. There is no papilloedema. Which one of the following is the diagnosis?

☐   A   *Haemophilus* meningitis

☐   B   Herpes simplex encephalitis

☐   C   Meningococcal meningitis

☐   D   Pneumococcal meningitis

☐   E   Tuberculous meningitis

2.34   A 76-year-old woman is brought to the clinic by her daughter. She is worried about her mother's increasing forgetfulness. Her mother has had increasing difficulty managing at home over several months, forgetting what she has bought and getting lost while out at the shops. The presence of which one of the following abnormalities lends most weight to a diagnosis of Alzheimer's disease?

☐   A   Constructional apraxia

☐   B   Disinhibition

☐   C   Disorientation in time

☐   D   Episodic memory deficit

☐   E   Visual hallucinations

2.35   A 32-year-old woman presents with choreiform movements and intellectual decline over a period of several years. She denies any family history of neurological disorder. On examination she has continual choreiform jerks involving the hands and feet; sensation, power and reflexes are normal, with flexor plantars. Which one of the following is the most likely diagnosis?

☐ A   Huntington's disease

☐ B   Multiple sclerosis

☐ C   Neuroacanthocytosis

☐ D   Parkinson's disease

☐ E   Wilson's disease

2.36   A 68-year-old female smoker complains of progressive difficulty with writing and simple mental arithmetic. On examination you find a lower right homonymous quadrantanopia; neuropsychological testing confirms a mild dyscalculia, dysgraphia and finger agnosia. You order an MRI scan; damage to which one of the following structures do you suspect is responsible for her symptoms?

☐ A   Left frontal lobe

☐ B   Left occipital lobe

☐ C   Left parietal lobe

☐ D   Right parietal lobe

☐ E   Left temporal lobe

2.37   A 34-year-old woman presents complaining of episodic leg weakness and crampy abdominal pain without diarrhoea. During an episode, her abdomen is distended with decreased bowel sounds, and she has distal leg weakness with loss of knee and ankle jerks. These findings suggest a defect in the biosynthetic pathway for:

☐ A   Collagen

☐ B   Corticosteroids

☐ C   Glucose

☐ D   Haem

☐ E   Thyroxine

2.38   A 24-year-old man presents with a seven-day history of progressive lower limb paraesthesiae, numbness extending from both feet up to the lower abdomen, and difficulty walking. Numbness has started to develop in his hands. You find generalised weakness and areflexia on examination, but without definite sensory loss. Which one of the following is the most likely diagnosis?

☐   A   Cervical cord compression

☐   B   Guillain–Barré syndrome

☐   C   Motor neurone disease

☐   D   Myasthenia gravis

☐   E   Polymyositis

2.39   A 26-year-old woman presents with two episodes of loss of consciousness. On each occasion she remembers a strong smell immediately before losing consciousness. Her work colleagues who observed these episodes report that she sat motionless at her desk, chewing repetitively for a few seconds, before slumping forwards. She was unconscious for about thirty seconds, subsequently appearing confused and disoriented for a few minutes. Physical examination, EEG and MRI are all normal. Which one of the following treatments is likely to be most appropriate?

☐   A   Carbamazepine

☐   B   Ethosuximide

☐   C   Gabapentin

☐   D   Lamotrigine

☐   E   Phenytoin

2.40   A 26-year-old woman is brought to the Emergency Department having collapsed in a nightclub with a tonic-clonic seizure. When you see her, she is awake and complaining of nausea and headache. On examination she has moderate pyramidal weakness of the right leg. A CT scan shows bilateral haemorrhagic infarction of the white matter in the left parietal lobe. The most likely cause is occlusion of which one of the following blood vessels?

☐   A   Cavernous sinus

☐   B   Left middle cerebral artery

☐   C   Left posterior cerebral artery

☐   D   Right anterior cerebral artery

☐   E   Sagittal sinus

2.41   A 34-year-old vegan presents with a six-week history of distressing paraesthesiae in the hands and legs. In the last two weeks, her gait has become unsteady and she feels her legs have become weak. On examination, vibration and joint-position sense is impaired in the lower limbs. Her legs show increased tone, a mild symmetrical proximal loss of power, hyper-reflexia and bilateral upgoing plantars. Her gait is ataxic. What nutritional deficiency is the likely cause of her problems?

☐ A   Folic acid

☐ B   Iron

☐ C   Pyridoxine

☐ D   Thiamine

☐ E   Vitamin B_{12}

2.42   A 29-year-old man presents with acute onset of wrist drop six weeks after breaking his leg. You find weakness of forearm extension, wrist and finger extension and loss of the triceps and brachioradialis reflexes, but with little sensory loss. Which one of the following branches of the brachial plexus is most likely to be affected?

☐ A   Axillary

☐ B   Dorsal scapular

☐ C   Median

☐ D   Radial

☐ E   Ulnar

2.43   A 52-year-old man has been suffering from progressive forgetfulness and unsteadiness of gait for two months. You observe spontaneous myoclonic twitching of his fingers, and elicit startle myoclonus to a loud noise. Neuropsychological examination reveals profound impairment of memory, attention and language function. Which one of the following is the most likely underlying diagnosis?

☐ A   Alzheimer's disease

☐ B   Creutzfeldt–Jakob disease

☐ C   Myoclonic epilepsy

☐ D   Pick's disease

☐ E   Subacute sclerosing panencephalitis

2.44 A 20-year-old man complains of an increasingly frequent irresistible urge to sleep several times a day, usually after a meal. After a brief nap he feels refreshed, but is increasingly disturbed that the episodes occur in embarrassing or unusual situations. He has occasionally experienced sudden weakness of the neck muscles and knees when laughing, sometimes causing him to fall to the floor. There are no neurological signs. What treatment is likely to be indicated?

☐ A   Adrenaline (epinephrine)

☐ B   Bromocriptine

☐ C   Dextroamphetamine

☐ D   Diazepam

☐ E   Imipramine

PSYCHIATRY

Best of Five

Questions

PSYCHIATRY: 'BEST OF FIVE' QUESTIONS

For each of the questions select the ONE most appropriate answer from the options provided.

3.1   A 30-year-old nurse has been referred to the clinic following a recent diagnosis of systemic lupus erythematosus (SLE). She feels she is having a 'nervous breakdown' and wishes to find out whether her SLE is affecting her mind. She is asking for advice on this matter. Which one of the following statements is most likely with regard to SLE and mental disorder?

☐ A   Cerebral manifestations occur in less than 10% of cases

☐ B   Schizophreniform psychosis is the commonest psychiatric manifestation

☐ C   Psychiatric symptoms are almost always due to cerebral arteritis

☐ D   Psychiatric symptoms usually precede fever and arthralgia

☐ E   Cerebral involvement is an indicator of poor prognosis

3.2   A 56-year-old man has been admitted following an episode of chest pain. He has a history of schizophrenia and has been on a depot antipsychotic for a number of years. You notice that he has quite marked abnormal involuntary movements. Movements include choreoathetosis and orofacial dyskinesia and you conclude he has tardive dyskinesia (TD). Which one of the following statements regarding tardive dyskinesia is most accurate?

☐ A   It is associated with previous brain damage

☐ B   It occurs in most patients on long-term neuroleptic treatment

☐ C   It is more common in men

☐ D   It is associated with reduced life expectancy in severe schizophrenia

☐ E   It invariably improves on stopping the offending neuroleptic

3.3   A 28-year-old woman has recently given birth to her first child. She
        presents to the Emergency Department complaining that the child is
        severely ill as he never stops crying. The child has been examined and does
        not appear to be unwell. However, you are concerned that the mother is
        exhibiting signs of mental disorder and may be in need of treatment. Which
        one of the following characteristics would most support a diagnosis of
        puerperal psychosis?

    ☐   A   Onset of symptoms within two days of the birth

    ☐   B   Onset of symptoms after two weeks from the birth

    ☐   C   Clouding of consciousness

    ☐   D   A past history of schizophrenia

    ☐   E   Despondency as the predominant underlying affective state

3.4   A 48-year-old man has been brought in by ambulance following a collapse
        in the street. He looks unkempt and smells strongly of alcohol. He is
        admitted to the ward for observation. The following day he has no
        recollection of how he passed out. You suspect he has a problem with
        alcohol and elicit an alcohol history. To determine the presence of alcohol
        dependence syndrome, which one of the following is least important with
        regard to making the diagnosis?

    ☐   A   A clear history of blackouts with cognitive deficits on assessment

    ☐   B   Altered tolerance to alcohol

    ☐   C   Drinking to relieve withdrawal symptoms

    ☐   D   Only drinking 9% lager from midday onwards

    ☐   E   A preference to stay drinking in the pub rather than to return home

3.5　A 47-year-old woman has been admitted to the ward in a severely dehydrated state. The history obtained from her husband is that his wife has been very depressed following the death of their only child. Over the past few weeks she has hardly been eating and is now refusing any fluids. An emergency course of electroconvulsive therapy (ECT) has been prescribed by the psychiatrists, under the provisions of the Mental Health Act. The husband is concerned about the ECT and asks you a number of questions regarding the treatment. Which one of his concerns regarding the proposed ECT is most valid?

- ☐ A　ECT can cause permanent damage to memory
- ☐ B　ECT can cause short-term memory loss
- ☐ C　Patients appear distressed during ECT, with arms and legs convulsing
- ☐ D　There is no good quality evidence demonstrating efficacy of ECT
- ☐ E　An antidepressant would be as effective as ECT for his wife and should be used in preference

3.6　A 48-year-old man frequently attends the clinic claiming that there has been no improvement in his symptoms despite several appropriate interventions. He does appear unhappy and you query whether he might be depressed. Which one of his following symptoms would most suggest a course of an antidepressant might lead to some improvement?

- ☐ A　Incongruity of mood and thinking
- ☐ B　Episodes of irritability and increased tempo of thought
- ☐ C　Improvement of mood every evening
- ☐ D　Chronic anhedonia
- ☐ E　Fluctuating levels of concentration

3.7   A 30-year-old woman presents with an exacerbation of long-standing asthma. She describes intermittent attacks of dyspnoea accompanied by prominent palpitations and tremor. She describes being very anxious during an attack and you query whether she has co-existing panic disorder which would benefit from treatment. The presence of which one of the following symptoms would add weight to the diagnosis of panic disorder?

- [ ] A   There is usually a clear precipitant to the attack
- [ ] B   There is an accompanying sense of impending doom
- [ ] C   Attacks last approximately one hour
- [ ] D   Staying as still as possible in one place helps the attack to subside
- [ ] E   The patient has underlying near-continuous feelings of nervousness in-between attacks

3.8   You are asked to see a 40-year-old man on a surgical ward who is complaining of atypical chest pain. He had an abdominal operation five days ago. The surgeons report clouding of consciousness for the first day post-op but none since. After assessing the patient you still suspect the patient may have an acute confusional state (delirium). Which one of the following features would be most consistent with this diagnosis?

- [ ] A   Abnormal psychomotor activity
- [ ] B   Autotopagnosia
- [ ] C   Catastrophic reaction
- [ ] D   Thought alienation
- [ ] E   Labile affect

3.9   A 29-year-old man has been admitted to the ward for a number of investigations for a renal complaint. He appears increasingly disruptive and has difficulty staying by his bedside. He is overfamiliar with staff and patients and is difficult to interrupt when you try and speak with him. Notes indicate that he has previously suffered from a mood disorder. You suspect he is becoming hypomanic. Which one of the following would be indicated as a first-line treatment to produce the most rapid improvement in his behaviour?

- [ ] A   Carbamazepine
- [ ] B   Electroconvulsive therapy (ECT)
- [ ] C   Lithium carbonate
- [ ] D   Olanzapine
- [ ] E   Procyclidine

3.10 Several days after admission for a chest infection, a 56-year-old man starts to complain that the nursing staff are deliberately harming him by administering poison rather than antibiotics. He refuses to take any more medication and you fear he will deteriorate. You reassess him and determine that he had been drinking alcohol excessively prior to admission. He was not treated for this and you suspect he has become mentally unwell as a result. He states voices have told him the nurses are against him. In trying to distinguish between alcoholic hallucinosis and delirium tremens, which one of the following would most support the former?

☐ A   Abnormal liver function tests

☐ B   A diagnosis of alcohol dependence syndrome

☐ C   Hallucinations in clear consciousness

☐ D   Insomnia

☐ E   Lilliputian hallucinations

3.11 You are reviewing a 46-year-old man in the Renal Clinic who is receiving chronic ambulatory peritoneal dialysis. He seems rather depressed and when asked, expresses hopelessness. You fear he might be a suicide risk and perform a risk assessment. The presence of which one of the following would most concern you with regard to urgent risk of suicide?

☐ A   Alcohol dependence

☐ B   Persistent thoughts that life is no longer worth living

☐ C   Schizophrenia

☐ D   Suicidal ideation

☐ E   Suicidal intent

3.12 A 15-year-old post-pubertal girl has been admitted in an emaciated state. She says she has lost her appetite because of the stress of taking examinations. She strongly denies being anorexic. Which one of the following from your assessment of her would lend most weight to a diagnosis of anorexia nervosa?

☐ A   A body mass index (BMI) of 16.5 kg/m^2

☐ B   A denial that she is underweight

☐ C   A previous history of bulimia nervosa

☐ D   Amenorrhoea

☐ E   Episodes of intermittent binge eating when unobserved

3.13 A 28-year-old man has been admitted having collapsed in the street. He refuses to speak to you. You suspect from his behaviour that he has a mental illness, but the patient denies this and you cannot access his GP out of hours. The only information you have is a list of his prescribed medication found by ambulance staff. In trying to distinguish which mental illness he may have, which one of the following of his medications would be least likely to be prescribed for a patient with schizo-affective disorder?

- ☐ A Chlordiazepoxide
- ☐ B Clozapine
- ☐ C Haloperidol
- ☐ D Procyclidine
- ☐ E Sodium valproate

3.14 You are reviewing a 46-year-old woman with multiple sclerosis in the clinic. Since starting on fluoxetine (a selective serotonin re-uptake inhibitor, SSRI) four months ago, her quality of life has improved and she no longer presents as feeling hopeless about the future. However, she states her antidepressant has given her a number of side-effects and she wishes to stop taking it. You attempt to reassure her that most of her symptoms are unlikely to be attributable to fluoxetine, except for which one of the following?

- ☐ A Anorgasmia
- ☐ B Extrapyramidal side-effects
- ☐ C Sedation
- ☐ D Suicidal thoughts
- ☐ E Withdrawal symptoms if she misses a dose

3.15 A 24-year-old man has been admitted following a life-threatening salicylate overdose. He has no past psychiatric history, although his mother states that over the past few months he has been behaving in an increasingly strange manner. The patient is initially unconscious. He subsequently develops a delirium with visual hallucinations. Several days later he appears to have recovered, but his hallucinations persist. In addition, he now appears to have some symptoms suggestive of schizophrenia. In order to determine whether there are organic factors contributing to his symptoms you organise an MRI brain scan. Which one of the following findings on his brain scan would be least likely to be attributable to schizophrenia?

☐ A   Cortical sulcal widening

☐ B   Lateral ventricular enlargement

☐ C   Reduced volume of medial temporal lobe structures

☐ D   Reduced volume of the third ventricle

☐ E   Widespread grey matter volume deficits

3.16 A 40-year-old man presents with rapidly progressing intellectual deterioration. You order a number of tests, including an electroencephalogram (EEG). Which one of the following EEG abnormalities would most likely be attributable to Creutzfeldt–Jakob disease (CJD)?

☐ A   Four-per-second spike-and-wave discharges

☐ B   Frontal intermittent rhythmic delta activity

☐ C   Generalised low-voltage fast activity or random slow activity, progressing to a flat record

☐ D   Low voltage with triphasic discharges

☐ E   Myoclonic flattening

3.17   A 48-year-old man has been referred for a medical opinion by his
        psychiatrist. The patient initially presented with treatment-resistant
        depression. He now presents with intellectual deterioration and abnormal
        involuntary movements. Having assessed him, you determine that the
        patient is not aware of any family history of a movement disorder. Despite
        this, you suspect Huntington's disease and order an MRI brain scan. Which
        one of the following abnormalities on a brain scan would provide most
        evidence for Huntington's disease?

    ☐   A   Basal ganglia atrophy
    ☐   B   Caudate atrophy
    ☐   C   Dilated ventricles
    ☐   D   Global atrophy
    ☐   E   Temporal lobe atrophy

3.18   You are reviewing a 35-year-old man with Down's syndrome at a yearly
        follow-up clinic for his cardiac problems. His carer accompanies him and
        states that the patient's behaviour has started to deteriorate and that he
        suspects a problem with his mental health. Which one of the following
        would be the most likely psychiatric cause?

    ☐   A   Alzheimer's dementia
    ☐   B   Temporolimbic epilepsy
    ☐   C   Manic depression
    ☐   D   Panic disorder
    ☐   E   Schizophrenia

3.19   A 56-year-old man being treated for Parkinson's disease has started to
        develop intrusive auditory hallucinations. You suspect levodopa has
        contributed to the development of psychosis. Despite reducing his
        medication, the hallucinations persist and you decide to start an
        antipsychotic. In considering an appropriate treatment which will not
        exacerbate the patient's parkinsonian symptoms, which one of the
        following antipsychotics has the least effect on D2 dopamine receptors?

    ☐   A   Chlorpromazine
    ☐   B   Haloperidol
    ☐   C   Quetiapine
    ☐   D   Risperidone
    ☐   E   Sulpiride

3.20 A 62-year-old female patient is acting bizarrely on the ward. After assessing her you believe she is not acutely confused but is psychotic. The presence of which one of the following would provide evidence that the patient is acutely psychotic?

- ☐ A Autochthonous delusions
- ☐ B Echopraxia
- ☐ C Hypnagogic hallucinations
- ☐ D Hypnapompic hallucinations
- ☐ E Tardive dyskinesia

3.21 You are called to the ward as the nursing staff are concerned that a 34-year-old male patient has been standing in the ward office for an hour and is refusing to move. You find that the patient is alert but unresponsive. You attempt to examine the patient. Which one of the following motor disturbances would most lead you to suspect catatonia?

- ☐ A Reduced tone
- ☐ B Catalepsy
- ☐ C Cataplexy
- ☐ D Stereotypy
- ☐ E Mannerisms

3.22 A 19-year-old man attends your clinic with his carer and is presenting with dyspnoea. The carer explains that the patient has learning difficulties but is unsure of the exact cause. Which one of the following would most support a diagnosis of fragile X syndrome?

- ☐ A Absence of male secondary sexual characteristics
- ☐ B Tall stature
- ☐ C Prognathism
- ☐ D Single palmar crease
- ☐ E Strabismus

3.23 A 24-year-old man presents complaining of unusually distributed chest pain. Following a careful assessment to exclude organic disorder, you decide he is suffering from somatic hallucinations. In trying to distinguish between schizophrenia and a drug-induced psychosis you take a history, looking at aetiological factors for his presentation. Which one of the following factors from his background is most associated with an increased risk of schizophrenia?

☐ A His nephew has been diagnosed with schizophrenia

☐ B He is Afro-Caribbean

☐ C He was born in the summer months

☐ D He is male

☐ E He has a history of childhood attention deficit disorder

3.24 A 28-year-old man has been referred following an overdose of 100 paracetamol tablets. Blood levels reveal a paracetamol level of zero. He also claims to have considerable abdominal pain but does not appear distressed, and physical examination reveals no abnormalities except for a number of abdominal scars. The patient is admitted to hospital for observation. Which one of the following would add most weight to a diagnosis of Munchausen's syndrome?

☐ A The prospect of financial gain from illness

☐ B The presence of alcohol dependence

☐ C The presence of secondary gain

☐ D Delusions of grandeur

☐ E Describing hearing unseen voices outside the patient's head

3.25 A 34-year-old man has been referred for an urgent medical opinion. He has been very agitated and has been treated with high doses of antipsychotics. The referring psychiatrist describes a number of clinical features which are suggestive of neuroleptic malignant syndrome. Which one of the following features is least compatible with this diagnosis?

☐ A Mutism

☐ B Dysphagia

☐ C Diaphoresis

☐ D Incontinence

☐ E Bradycardia

3.26   A 24-year-old man, recently admitted to a medical ward, now discloses that he is a heroin addict. He is demanding that you help alleviate his withdrawal symptoms – otherwise he will self-discharge. There are no contraindications to a pharmacological approach. Which one of the following would you consider the most appropriate to treat his withdrawal symptoms?

☐ A   Bupropion

☐ B   Chlorpromazine

☐ C   Diamorphine

☐ D   Lofexidine

☐ E   Oxazepam

3.27   A 30-year-old woman presents claiming her heart is failing. You find no abnormalities on physical examination but you elicit a number of abnormalities on mental state examination. The presence of which one of the following abnormalities lends most weight to a diagnosis of schizophrenia?

☐ A   Catatonia

☐ B   Gustatory hallucinations

☐ C   Primary delusion

☐ D   Neologisms

☐ E   Tangential responses to questioning

3.28   A 22-year-old woman of Indian origin is admitted as an emergency because of dehydration and very low body weight. She gives a long history of low weight, poor appetite and frequent nausea and vomiting. Which one of the following would make you most likely to suspect a diagnosis of anorexia nervosa?

☐ A   Acknowledgement of being severely underweight

☐ B   Avoidance of Western food

☐ C   Body mass index (BMI) of 17 kg/m^2

☐ D   Minimal appetite

☐ E   Self-induced vomiting

3.29 A 57-year-old married man with chronic renal failure describes poor energy levels and disturbed sleep. He goes on to describe anhedonia, guilt and hopelessness and appears unhappy. You believe he is depressed. The patient will not consider antidepressants, but agrees to talk to a therapist. Which one of the following psychological treatments is likely to be most effective?

- ☐ A Cognitive behavioural therapy
- ☐ B Family therapy
- ☐ C Psychoanalysis
- ☐ D Psychodynamic therapy
- ☐ E Supportive therapy

3.30 You are reviewing a 26-year-old woman with poorly controlled diabetes. She attends appointments erratically and you decide compliance should be optimised. In considering reasons for poor attendance, which one of the following would lead you to think agoraphobia was a possible reason?

- ☐ A Anxiety in crowded places
- ☐ B Anxiety in enclosed spaces
- ☐ C Anxiety in social situations
- ☐ D Free-floating anxiety
- ☐ E Unpredictable panic attacks

3.31 A 38-year-old colleague complains of being under considerable stress at work and fears that he is becoming mentally unwell. He describes a number of recent unusual experiences. Which one of the following would most lead you to suspect the presence of a psychotic disorder?

- ☐ A Depersonalisation
- ☐ B Derealisation
- ☐ C Hypnagogic hallucinations
- ☐ D Hypnapompic hallucinations
- ☐ E Thought alienation

3.32   A 19-year-old man admitted four days ago appears to be experiencing
auditory hallucinations and thought broadcasting and has expressed
persecutory delusions to the nursing staff. His girlfriend admits he has
experimented with a drug of abuse prior to admission. Which one of the
following drugs is most likely to produce a schizophreniform psychosis?

☐ A   Amphetamine

☐ B   Cannabis

☐ C   Heroin

☐ D   LSD

☐ E   Psilocybin

3.33   You are reviewing a 56-year-old woman with angina in the clinic. She was
widowed one month ago and you are concerned about the state of her
mental health. Which one of the following would make you most
concerned that this lady is demonstrating pathological grief?

☐ A   Inability to feel sadness

☐ B   Intense yearning for her dead husband

☐ C   Loss of appetite

☐ D   Poor sleep

☐ E   Visions of her dead husband

3.34   A 30-year-old male political refugee has been attending hospital for several
months complaining of abdominal pains. Despite extensive investigations,
no organic cause has been identified. Further history-taking leads you to
query the relevance of possible psychological factors. Which one of the
following features would most support a diagnosis of post-traumatic stress
disorder (PTSD)?

☐ A   Believing his persecutors have followed him to the UK

☐ B   Diurnal variation of mood

☐ C   Early-morning wakening

☐ D   Intrusive flashbacks

☐ E   Panic attacks

3.35 A 78-year-old lady recently diagnosed with dementia appears to you to be depressed. You take a history and then perform a cognitive and mental state examination. Which one of the following abnormalities is most likely to make you consider a diagnosis of depressive pseudodementia rather than dementia?

☐ A   Global memory loss

☐ B   Good effort at testing

☐ C   Poor concentration

☐ D   Poor historian

☐ E   Topographical disorientation

3.36 A 45-year-old lady has been complaining of multiple, varying gastrointestinal symptoms for three years. Despite extensive investigations and second opinions, she refuses to accept that there is no physical explanation for her symptoms. She complains her life has been completely disrupted because of her symptoms and wants more tests to seek an answer. From the information given, which one of the following diagnoses is most appropriate?

☐ A   Conversion disorder

☐ B   Dissociative disorder

☐ C   Hypochondriacal disorder

☐ D   Hysterical disorder

☐ E   Somatisation disorder

3.37 Which one of the following is the most common psychiatric complication in multiple sclerosis?

☐ A   Euphoria

☐ B   Intellectual deterioration

☐ C   Major depressive episode

☐ D   Psychotic episode

☐ E   Suicide

3.38   A 26-year-old primigravida has been referred urgently by her GP. The GP's letter states that she has had persistent, recurrent vomiting. Her appetite has been poor and she has eaten very little for several weeks. The GP's letter also states that she has been appearing increasingly confused. Cognitive examination reveals clear consciousness, temporal disorientation, intact registration and impaired five-minute recall. With regard to the cognitive deficits, what is the most likely diagnosis?

- ☐   A   Acute organic brain syndrome
- ☐   B   Creutzfeldt–Jakob disease
- ☐   C   Frontal lobe syndrome
- ☐   D   Korsakoff's syndrome
- ☐   E   Pre-senile dementia

3.39   A mother accompanies her 30-year-old son to the clinic. He has been referred for poor energy levels and fatigue. You discover that he has previously been treated for schizophrenia but no longer attends psychiatric follow-up. Assessment and investigations reveal no obvious cause for lethargy and you suspect the patient may be suffering negative symptoms of schizophrenia. Which one of the following is not a feature of negative schizophrenia?

- ☐   A   Alogia
- ☐   B   Anhedonia
- ☐   C   Avolition
- ☐   D   Blunting of affect
- ☐   E   Negativism

3.40   A 74-year-old man has been referred to you, as over the past few weeks his behaviour has been becoming increasingly bizarre. As part of your assessment you perform a cognitive examination. Which one of the following abnormalities is most suggestive of frontal lobe dysfunction?

- ☐   A   Hypersomnia
- ☐   B   Impaired five-minute recall
- ☐   C   Perseverating responses
- ☐   D   Right-left disorientation
- ☐   E   Sensory dysphasia

3.41 **Which one of the following conditions is least likely to concern you with regard to suicide risk?**

☐ A Chronic renal failure

☐ B Obsessive-compulsive disorder

☐ C Opiate dependence

☐ D Peptic ulcer disease

☐ E Schizophrenia

3.42 **A 32-year-old man with no known history of mental illness presents in a highly agitated state. He appears to be experiencing distressing hallucinations and persecutory delusions. His behaviour is becoming increasingly aggressive and is no longer manageable. Which one of the following would be the most appropriate initial pharmacological intervention?**

☐ A Intramuscular chlorpromazine

☐ B Intramuscular diazepam

☐ C Intramuscular haloperidol

☐ D Intramuscular lorazepam

☐ E Intravenous haloperidol

3.43 **A 38-year-old man admitted after a fall continues to complain of memory loss one week after the injury. At the ward round, dissociative amnesia is queried as a possibility. Which one of the following features would most strongly support this diagnosis?**

☐ A Fluctuating awareness

☐ B Fluctuating consciousness

☐ C Fluctuating recall

☐ D Predominant distress

☐ E Temporal disorientation

3.44 A 33-year-old woman's behaviour on an inpatient ward is becoming increasingly unusual. She appears to be overinvolved with other patients' management and reacts irritably when requested to return to her bed by staff. Nurses also report she has had very little sleep or food and that her speech makes little sense. After speaking to the patient, you agree that her speech is difficult to comprehend and suspect a manic episode. Which one of the following descriptions of speech lends additional weight to the diagnosis?

- [ ] A   Sentences include overly detailed descriptions of events
- [ ] B   Sentences spoken are connected by clanging
- [ ] C   Sentences spoken are connected obliquely
- [ ] D   There is repetition of a phrase several times
- [ ] E   There is sudden stopping of speech mid-sentence, followed by a new thought

3.45 A 29-year-old man refuses to undress and lie on a couch for a physical examination. He states that the couch is dirty and that he does not want to risk getting an infection. Which one of the following features would most lead you to suspect a diagnosis of obsessive-compulsive disorder?

- [ ] A   Acknowledging that this belief is irrational, but still refusing
- [ ] B   Believing that all hospital couches are contaminated by bacteria and are an infection risk
- [ ] C   Having a panic attack when approaching the couch
- [ ] D   Hearing a voice telling him the couch is infected
- [ ] E   Performing an elaborate, enjoyable prayer ritual before undressing

3.46 One year after a severe head injury, which one of the following cognitive deficits is most likely to be present?

- [ ] A   Disorder of executive functioning
- [ ] B   Fluent dysphasia
- [ ] C   Non-fluent dysphasia
- [ ] D   Non-verbal IQ loss
- [ ] E   Short-term memory loss

3.47 A patient on long-term lithium treatment for prophylaxis of bipolar affective disorder is complaining of feeling unwell. You wish to exclude lithium toxicity as a possible diagnosis. Which one of the following abnormalities is most likely to indicate toxicity?

☐ A Ataxia

☐ B Diarrhoea

☐ C Metallic taste

☐ D Oedema

☐ E Tremor

3.48 A General Practitioner has finally referred a 49-year-old woman to your clinic for long-standing weakness of her left arm. The GP confirms that this symptom has been present for three years. Following your assessment, you suspect a motor conversion disorder. Which one of the following features would not lend weight to the diagnosis?

☐ A A state of indifference to the paralysis

☐ B An obvious precipitant

☐ C Fasciculations

☐ D Muscle wasting

☐ E Significant secondary gain

3.49 A 24-year-old woman has been brought to hospital after collapsing. She appears physically well but says she has not been eating much. You suspect an eating disorder may have contributed to her presentation and take a detailed history. Which one of the following statements would not be true of bulimia nervosa?

☐ A Compensatory behaviour to counteract the fattening effect of food must be present

☐ B There are frequent episodes of fasting

☐ C There are overvalued ideas of shape/weight

☐ D There is a loss of control over eating

☐ E The majority of cases are preceded by anorexia nervosa

3.50 **Nursing staff report that a recently admitted inpatient has been complaining of hearing voices. He has a known history of alcohol dependence syndrome. Which one of the following features would most support a diagnosis of alcoholic hallucinosis?**

- ☐ A Hallucinations appear as part of an alcohol withdrawal syndrome
- ☐ B Hallucinations are not generally distressing
- ☐ C Hallucinations are third-person auditory
- ☐ D Hallucinations continue for more than six months
- ☐ E Hallucinations must occur in clear consciousness

BASIC SCIENCES: 'BEST OF FIVE' ANSWERS

1.1   C: All his offspring have a 50% chance of inheriting the disease

Huntington's disease is an autosomal dominant disorder, ie it results from mutation of one copy (allele) of a gene carried on an autosome. There is full penetrance so all individuals with the genetic mutation manifest the disease. The gene affected is on chromosome 4 and produces a protein called huntingtin. Within this gene there is expansion of the CAG trinucleotide repeat. Other trinucleotide repeat disorders include: myotonic dystrophy, fragile X syndrome, Friedriech's ataxia, spinocerebellar atrophy, spinobulbar muscular atrophy.

In normal individuals the number of trinucleotide repeats varies slightly but remains below a defined threshold. Affected patients have expansion above the disease-causing threshold. The length of the expansion increases as cells divide throughout life (somatic instability) and corresponds with the age of onset of disease. The expansions enlarge further in successive generations, causing increased disease severity and earlier onset (anticipation).

Onset of Huntington's usually occurs in the third or fourth decade. Patients usually present with chorea (a continuous flow of jerky movements from limb to limb) and cognitive decline. There is usually a positive family history. Other presenting symptoms include dysarthria, dysphagia, ataxia, myoclonus and dystonia. Childhood onset is atypical and may be associated with rigidity. Neuropathologically, the disease causes neuronal loss in the cortex and striatum, especially in the caudate nucleus. Treatment is unsatisfactory and doesn't prevent progression. Neuroleptics may help reduce chorea by inhibiting dopaminergic transmission. Death usually occurs 10 to 20 years after disease onset. Genetic testing and counselling is available for patients and asymptomatic relatives.

**1.2   E: When both parents carry the gene each of their offspring has a 25%
        chance of being affected and a 50% chance of being a carrier**

Wilson's disease is an autosomal recessive disorder with a gene frequency of 1 in 400 and a disease prevalence of approximately 1 in 200 000. The responsible gene is on chromosome 13 and codes for a copper-transporting ATPase. Autosomal recessive disorders result from mutations in both copies (alleles) of an autosomal gene. Both sexes are usually equally affected. Heterozygotes are carriers.

1.3   D: It allows specific DNA sequences to be amplified from a single cell

The polymerase chain reaction is an amplification reaction in which a small amount of DNA (the template) is amplified to produce enough to perform analysis. Two oligonucleotide primers are mixed with a DNA template and a thermostable DNA polymerase (Taq polymerase) derived from *T. aquaticus*, an organism that inhabits thermal springs. The mixture is heated to just below 100 °C and the DNA dissociates into two single strands. As the mixture cools, the oligonucleotide primers bind to either side of the specific area of interest in the DNA. The reaction is heated to 72 °C for about a minute and the DNA polymerase catalyses the synthesis of a copy of the DNA between the two primers. The process can be repeated many times to make multiple copies of the gene of interest. PCR is extremely powerful: to detect a given sequence of DNA it only needs to be present in one copy, ie one molecule of DNA.

Clinical applications of PCR include:

- mutation detection
- detection of viral and bacterial sequences in tissue (eg TB, HSV, hepatitis C, HIV)
- prenatal diagnosis, from chorionic villus sampling, of known genetic mutations, eg cystic fibrosis, Duchenne muscular dystrophy
- PCR of *in vitro* fertilised embryo to diagnose genetic disease before implantation
- forensic medicine.

Reverse transcription PCR enables us to investigate what genes in the total genome are expressed. It does this by amplifying those genes that are being transcribed into messenger RNA (mRNA).

RNA is too unstable to be used in PCR: it needs to be converted to complementary DNA (cDNA) using reverse transcriptase. This retroviral enzyme makes a precise copy of mRNA. PCR is then performed in the usual way. Because the template reflects the mRNA of the starting material, this technique can look at gene expression in individual tissues. Clinical applications of reverse transcription PCR include:

- basic scientific research into the normal function of genes by understanding their expression
- detection of the expression of particular genes in tumour tissue
- detection of RNA viruses in tissue.

Stem E describes Southern blotting, a technique used to detect and determine the size of specific restriction fragments in DNA, and hence detect a specific gene of interest.

1.4   C: The left coronary artery usually bifurcates into the left anterior descending (LAD) artery and the circumflex artery

The right coronary artery usually arises from the anterior aortic sinus and the left from the posterior aortic cusp. The right coronary artery usually supplies the AV node. Either the right or the left coronary artery may supply the sinoatrial (SA) node. The right coronary artery gives off a posterior descending branch.

1.5   E: Paralysis of the thenar muscles, ie opponens pollicis, abductor pollicis brevis and flexor pollicis brevis

The median nerve arises from the lateral and medial cords of the brachial plexus (C6–8, T1) and sends a motor supply to:

* the lateral two lumbricals (L)
* opponens pollicis (O), abductor pollicis brevis (A) and flexor pollicis brevis (F), ie the thenar eminence muscles
* all the muscles on the flexor aspect of the forearm apart from flexor carpi ulnaris and the ulnar half of the flexor digitorum profundus.

It supplies sensation to the palmar aspect of the thumb and the lateral two and a half fingers. Median nerve damage at the wrist causes paralysis and wasting of the thenar muscles. Median nerve damage at the elbow also causes ulnar deviation and weak wrist flexion. Pronation of the forearm is lost. The signs described in stems A, B and C are features of ulnar nerve damage. Wrist drop is caused by damage to the radial nerve.

1.6   D: A temporal lobe lesion

Lesions at the optic radiation in the temporal lobe result in a contralateral homonymous hemianopia. Lesions at the optic chiasma typically produce a bitemporal hemianopia. A lesion in the right parietal lobe would result in a contralateral inferior quadrantanopia. Posterior cerebral artery occlusion tends to produce a contralateral homonymous hemianopia with macular sparing. (The macular region of the occipital cortex is on the tip of the occipital lobe, a vascular watershed area supplied by the posterior and middle cerebral arteries. Therefore it may be spared when a posterior cerebral artery CVA occurs.) Optic neuritis typically causes an ipsilateral central scotoma.

1.7   E: Metoclopramide

Galactorrhoea is caused by excess prolactin secretion. Prolactin release from the pituitary is under negative control by dopamine from the hypothalamus. Therefore dopamine and dopamine agonists, like bromocriptine, reduce prolactin release. Dopamine antagonists (such as metoclopramide) increase prolactin release.

Other causes of hyperprolactinaemia and galactorrhoea are:

• pregnancy

• stress, eg epileptic fit

• oestrogens (oral contraceptive pill)

• phenothiazines (like metoclopramide, are dopamine antagonists)

• damage to the hypothalamus or pituitary stalk, eg by radiation or tumour

• renal or hepatic failure

• nipple stimulation

• polycystic ovarian syndrome.

1.8   C: It is contraindicated in Wolff–Parkinson–White syndrome

Digoxin is a sodium/potassium ATPase inhibitor. It slows conduction through the AV node and is therefore used to control ventricular rate in atrial tachycardias and fibrillation. It is also positively inotropic and is used to treat heart failure, where it has been shown to improve symptoms and hospitalisation rates but not mortality.

WPW syndrome is associated with an accessory pathway connecting the atrium and ventricle. Conduction along this accessory pathway can mediate a narrow-complex tachycardia and can also predispose to unopposed conduction of atrial fibrillation to the ventricle. Digoxin can accelerate conduction down the accessory pathway by blocking the AV node and therefore should be avoided.

Digoxin is also contraindicated in complete heart block, second degree heart block, and hypertrophic cardiomyopathy. Digoxin has a number of adverse effects, including: arrhythmias, heart block, nausea and vomiting, diarrhoea, headache, confusion, visual disturbance (xanthopsia, yellow vision), and gynaecomastia.

Digoxin toxicity may be enhanced by electrolyte abnormalities (hypokalaemia, hypomagnesaemia and hypercalcaemia), renal impairment and interaction with other drugs. Life-threatening toxicity can be treated with Fab fragment antibody specific for digoxin (Digibind®). 'Reversed tick' ST-segment depression is commonly seen in the inferior and lateral leads on the ECG, and represents a sign of digoxin therapy and not specifically digoxin toxicity.

1.9   E: Amiodarone toxicity

The patient has biochemical evidence of hepatitis and hyperthyroidism. His PFTs suggest a restrictive deficit with decreased transfer factor. In a patient who has been attending the Cardiology Clinic for several years and who has underlying atrial fibrillation, it is highly likely that these abnormalities are due to amiodarone toxicity.

Amiodarone is a class III antiarrhythmic which is very effective in the management of supraventricular and ventricular tachycardia. It is, however, associated with several side-effects and complications:

- hyper- or hypothyroidism
- photosensitivity
- hepatitis
- peripheral neuropathy
- pulmonary fibrosis
- corneal microdeposits
- metallic taste in the mouth
- skin discoloration (slate-grey pigmentation)
- arrhythmias
- ataxia
- optic neuritis
- myopathy
- epididymitis
- nausea.

CCF is unlikely. Although right heart failure may cause hepatitis, and pulmonary oedema secondary to left-sided failure may cause a restrictive deficit and reduced transfer factor, CCF is unlikely in view of the echo. Also, this answer does not satisfactorily explain the patient's hyperthyroidism and skin discoloration. A chest infection would not account for the skin discoloration, blood tests or PFTs. Hyperthyroidism would not explain the patient's breathlessness, skin discoloration, hepatitis or PFTs. Hereditary haemochromatosis is an autosomal recessive disorder of iron metabolism, in which increased iron absorption leads to its deposition in multiple organs. It can cause bronze or slate-grey skin pigmentation, hepatitis, hepatomegaly and cirrhosis. In the heart it may cause a dilated cardiomyopathy and arrhythmias. It does not account for this patient's hyperthyroidism or PFTs.

1.10 E: Pituitary insufficiency

This lady has hypoglycaemia. Polycystic ovarian syndrome is associated with insulin resistance and therefore patients are more likely to develop diabetes mellitus (DM) or impaired glucose tolerance. In haemochromatosis, iron may accumulate in the pancreas, leading to insulin deficiency and secondary diabetes. Steroid therapy causes insulin resistance and thereby diabetes and impaired glucose tolerance.

Metformin does not cause cause hypoglycaemia. Fasting hypoglycaemia may be caused by administration of insulin/sulphonylureas, insulinoma, alcohol (alcohol metabolism occurs at the expense of hepatic gluconeogenesis), Addison's disease, pituitary insufficiency (due to impaired growth hormone and ACTH secretion), liver failure, non-pancreatic tumours (especially retroperitoneal sarcomas), or autoimmune hypoglycaemia (eg in Hodgkin's disease). Insulin receptor antibodies normally cause insulin-resistant DM by blocking the insulin receptor. Rarely they cause receptor activation with fasting hypoglycaemia. Anti-insulin antibodies cause accumulation of antibody-bound insulin, which then dissociates, resulting in high insulin levels. Post-prandial hypoglycaemia can occur post-gastrectomy.

1.11 E: Porphyria cutanea tarda

The porphyrias are a group of inherited disorders that result from deficiency of one of the enzymes in the haem synthetic pathway. Porphyria cutanea tarda (PCT) is the commonest form of porphyria. It is usually only expressed in the presence of hepatic damage, usually from another cause (particularly alcohol). Clinical features include photosensitivity, blisters, scarring, hyperpigmentation and hypertrichosis. It is caused by reduced uroporphyrinogen decarboxylase activity. Uroporphyrinogen accumulates in blood and urine in acute attacks. In remission there is excess porphyrin in the faeces. Treatment comprises treatment of underlying liver disease, venesection and chloroquine.

1.12 E: Ethanol toxicity

This patient has a high anion gap acidosis. She also has a raised osmolal gap. The osmolal gap is the difference between the lab estimation of osmolality and the calculated osmolality. To calculate the plasma osmolality:

$$2([Na^+]+[K^+]) + [urea] + [glucose]$$

The osmolal gap is usually < 10. If it is > 10 consider: raised levels of alcohol, eg methanol, ethanol, ethylene glycol, isopranolol, diethyleneglycol; diabetes mellitus; renal failure (retention of various organic and inorganic molecules).

Type 2 RTA and Addison's disease are associated with normal anion gap acidosis.

Salicylate toxicity gives a high anion gap acidosis but doesn't produce a high osmolal gap. Conn's syndrome causes a metabolic alkalosis.

1.13   D: Conn's syndrome

This patient has a metabolic alkalosis. Renal failure and Addison's disease cause a metabolic acidosis. Anxiety may be associated with hyperventilation, which may cause a respiratory alkalosis. Salicylate poisoning causes a respiratory alkalosis and metabolic acidosis.

Causes of a metabolic alkalosis are:

1. Acid loss:
    *   gastrointestinal tract – vomiting, nasogastric aspiration, antacids (in renal failure)
    *   renal – diuretics, mineralocorticoids (Conn's, Cushing's), chronic hypercapnia, Bartter's syndrome, hypercalcaemia
    *   cellular – hypokalaemia
2. Bicarbonate addition – blood transfusions (citrate), sodium bicarbonate treatment, milk-alkali syndrome
3. Contraction (loss of chloride-rich/bicarbonate-poor fluid) – diuretics, diarrhoea and vomiting.

1.14   B: Alkaptonuria

This is a rare autosomal recessive disease. Homogentisic acid accumulates as a result of a deficiency in the enzyme homogentisic acid oxidase. The homogentisic acid polymerises to produce the black-brown alkapton, which is deposited in cartilage and connective tissue. Urine becomes dark on standing due to oxidation and polymerisation of homogentisic acid. Abnormal pigmentation is found in the ear and sclerae as well as articular cartilage. Premature arthritis occurs, predominantly affecting the spine, and later the large joints. Intervertebral disc calcification is characteristic of alkaptonuria. The knees are commonly affected, although there is usually sparing of the sacroiliac joints. The diagnosis is confirmed by checking a urinary homogentisic acid level. Homogentisic acid is a reducing substance and therefore gives a positive reaction to glucostix (Clinistix). Other causes of false-positive results are: fructose, pentose, lactose, salicylates, ascorbic acid.

1.15 B: Severe diarrhoea

This question is about the anion gap. The normal anion gap is 12–16 mmol/l and represents unmeasured anions present on fixed or organic acids, eg albumin, phosphate, sulphate, lactate and ketones.

The anion gap = $(Na^+ + K^+) - (Cl^- + HCO_3^-)$

In high anion gap acidosis, the decreased bicarbonate (due to buffering/titration of hydrogen ion) reflects the accumulation of unmeasured acid anions.

Causes of an increased anion gap include: lactic acidosis, ketoacidosis (secondary to alcohol or diabetes mellitus), renal failure, drugs/toxins (salicylates, biguanides, ethylene glycol, methanol).

Normal anion gap acidosis occurs where there is loss of bicarbonate or ingestion of hydrogen ion. Chloride is retained. Causes include: renal tubular acidosis type 1 and 2, drugs (acetazolamide), Addison's disease, pancreatic or biliary fistulae, severe diarrhoea, ureteric diversion, ammonium chloride ingestion.

1.16 C: Type 1 (distal) renal tubular acidosis (RTA)

This patient has a hypokalaemic hyperchloraemic normal anion gap acidosis. Despite the severe systemic acidosis she has not acidified her urine. She has also had two vertebral crush fractures, an unusual occurrence without prior trauma in someone so young. In the context of the history it may suggest the presence of osteoporosis. The right loin pain suggests urinary tract infection or calculus.

Type 1 RTA is typically severe (the bicarbonate may be reduced below 10 mmol/l). The basic defect is an inability to secrete protons in the distal tubule. This results in an inappropriate inability to acidify the urine below 5.3. Since H^+ reabsorption is abnormal, more sodium is reabsorbed, either with chloride or in exchange for potassium to maintain electroneutrality (hence the hyperchloraemia and hypokalaemia). Complications include osteoporosis, nephrocalcinosis and renal calculi. Growth failure and urinary tract infections may also occur. A renal calculus may be present, but this answer doesn't account for the history of fractures, the serum biochemistry and urinary pH.

DKA doesn't cause a normal anion gap acidodis and wouldn't lead to failure to acidify the urine. This answer also doesn't tie in with the history of vertebral fractures.

A UTI may cause these symptoms and haematuria but doesn't expain the fractures, urinary pH or serum biochemistry.

Type 2 (proximal) RTA typically causes a less severe acidosis (with a bicarbonate of 14–20 mmol/l). It causes osteomalacia and rickets rather than osteoporosis (due to phosphate wasting and reduced production of 1,25-dihydroxy D_3. The basic defect is proximal tubular bicarbonate wasting due to a resetting of the T_{max} of bicarbonate reabsorption. In the stable state bicarbonate wasting does not persist as the plasma bicarbonate stabilises at the concentration at which the proximal tubule is able to absorb all the filtered bicarbonate. Therefore the urine is typically appropriately acidified, especially in the morning. There may be other tubular abnormalities, such as glycosuria, aminoaciduria, uricosuria and phosphaturia.

1.17　D: Acute intermittent porphyria

Acute intermittent porphyria (AIP) is a porphyria, one of the hereditary disorders resulting from deficiency of one of the enzymes in the haem synthetic pathway. In AIP there is reduced porphobilinogen deaminase activity. It is autosomal dominant. Females are affected more than males. Clinical features include abdominal pain, vomiting and constipation; peripheral neuropathies (mainly motor); hypertension and tachycardia (secondary to autonomic neuropathy); convulsions and psychiatric disturbance. It can be associated with fever, papilloedema, raised WCC and ESR and hyponatraemia (due to SIADH). There is no photosensitivity or skin rash.

Precipitants include stress, infection and female hormones. Drug precipitants include alcohol, benzodiazepines, rifampicin, oral contraceptives, phenytoin and sulphonamides. Investigations reveal elevated δ aminolaevulinic acid (δALA) and porphobilinogen (PBG) in the urine and serum. Red cell PBG deaminase is reduced and δALA synthetase is increased. Treatment comprises avoidance of precipitants, high carbohydrate intake, haem arginine and supportive management.

1.18　B: Chronic liver disease occurs in 50–80% of those infected

Hepatitis C is an RNA virus. Interferon-α results in clearance of the virus in only 25% of patients with chronic liver disease. It initially leads to normalisation of liver function and loss of HCV RNA in 50% of patients, although six months later 50% of these are positive again. Ribavirin is also used to treat chronic infection. Fulminant hepatitis is very rare. Transmission is by sexual contact or through contaminated blood.

1.19   E: It may be transmitted by corneal grafts

Creutzfeldt–Jakob disease (CJD) is a transmissible spongiform encephalopathy. It is caused by a prion protein. Prions are glycoproteins derived from a gene (*PrP*) on chromosome 20 that codes for a normal membrane protein whose function is unclear. In prion diseases a modified form of this protein accumulates in neurones and neuropil, forming plaques and causing vacuolation of neurones (spongiform change). Prion proteins are not destroyed by proteolytic enzymes, heat ionising radiation, DNAase, RNAase, formaldehyde or disinfectants.

CJD may be :

- genetic – caused by an inherited genetic mutation in the prion protein gene
- iatrogenic – has been caused by corneal grafts, the use of infected dural grafts in neurosurgery, human cadaveric growth hormone and pituitary gonadotrophin
- sporadic – unknown cause
- variant – due to infection with the same prion protein that causes bovine spongiform encephalopathy in cattle; probably transmitted via contaminated food.

The clinical progression of sporadic CJD is usually very rapid. The median life expectancy is four months. CT head scans are usually normal in sporadic CJD, although sometimes atrophy is seen, particularly with illness of long duration.

Diagnosis is made on the basis of:

- the clinical history and examination findings
- EEG – typically generalised biphasic or triphasic periodic sharp-wave complexes appear with a frequency of 1 or 2 per second
- CSF analysis – elevated 14-3-3 protein (low specificity for CJD)
- MRI.

The definitive diagnosis is made by neuropathological examination of brain tissue.

1.20   D: Blood levels of HBeAg correlate with infectivity

HbeAg and HBV DNA correlate with viral replication, and hence infectivity. The virus may be found in cell types other than hepatocytes, eg renal tubules, lymph nodes. This may partly explain recurrence after transplantation. Approximately 10% develop chronic infection. IgG HbcAb alone implies continuing viral replication. IgG HbcAb in low titres, together with HBsAb implies a previous, cleared infection. Patients who are immunodeficient are more likely to develop chronic viral hepatitis than those who are immunocompetent. Successful clearance of the virus is dependent on the cell-mediated immune response. The stronger the response, the more cells die and the higher the enzyme levels. The opposite occurs in immunocompromised patients. They are more likely to develop chronic disease.

1.21 E: Severe complications occur due to the production of an exotoxin that inhibits protein synthesis

This patient has diphtheria. This is caused by infection with *Corynebacterium diphtheriae*, an aerobic, non-invasive Gram-positive rod. The organism produces an exotoxin that inhibits protein synthesis and causes local tissue destruction and membrane formation. It affects all cells but its most prominent effects are seen in the heart (where it causes myocarditis), nerves (where it leads to demyelination) and kidneys (where it produces tubular necrosis). Disease may involve almost any mucous membrane. The most common sites of infection are the pharynx and tonsils. Patients usually present with malaise, a sore throat, anorexia and a low-grade fever. Within two to three days a membrane forms and extends. The larynx may be involved, leading to hoarseness, a barking cough and, in some cases, airway obstruction.

Severe complications are due to the toxin. The severity of these is usually proportional to the severity of the local disease. Myocarditis may lead to heart failure and arrhythmias. Neurological complications mainly affect motor nerves. Local paralysis with paralysis of the soft palate and involvement of other cranial nerves may occur in the first few days. A peripheral neuritis, principally motor, may occur later. This usually begins proximally and extends distally. Respiratory failure and pneumonia may result. Treatment should be begun as soon as a presumptive diagnosis is made. This consists of diphtheria antitoxin, erythromycin, isolation and supportive management. Close contacts should receive prophylactic antibiotics and a diphtheria booster.

1.22 D: An overdose of diazepam

The patient in the question has type II respiratory failure: hypoxia ($PaO_2 < 8$ kPa) with a raised $PaCO_2$ (> 6.5 kPa). Type II respiratory failure results from alveolar hypoventilation with or without ventilation/perfusion (V/Q) mismatch.
Causes include:

- thoracic wall disease, eg kyphoscoliosis, flail chest, ankylosing spondylitis
- neurological disorders, eg Guillain–Barré, multiple sclerosis, polio, motor neurone disease, cervical cord lesion
- muscular disease, eg myasthenia gravis, muscular dystrophy
- sedative drugs
- pulmonary disease, eg COPD, late stages of severe asthma, emphysema, pulmonary fibrosis.

Type I respiratory failure is defined as hypoxia ($PaO_2 < 8$ kPa) with a low or normal $PaCO_2$. It is caused primarily by V/Q mismatch. Causes of type I respiratory failure include: pulmonary embolism, pneumonia, asthma, pulmonary oedema, pulmonary haemorrhage, pneumothorax, adult respiratory distress syndrome, fibrosing alveolitis, emphysema.

1.23   A: An increase in the pH

A rise in the pH shifts the oxygen-haemoglobin dissociation curve to the left. An increase in the hydrogen ion concentration shifts it to the right. When the curve is shifted to the right, haemoglobin gives up oxygen. This situation occurs in working or stressed muscle where there is:

* a rise in CO_2 due to increased metabolism
* a rise in hydrogen ion concentration (ie a fall in pH)
* an increase in temperature
* an increase in lactate production.

It also occurs in chronic hypoxic states and in chronic anaemia (which causes an increase in red blood cell 2,3-diphosphoglycerate).

The oxygen-haemoglobin dissociation curve is shifted to the left by the changes opposite to those above, and by haemoglobins with high oxygen affinities. These include carboxyhaemoglobin, methaemoglobin, sulfhaemoglobin and fetal haemoglobin.

1.24   D: Increased protein synthesis

Insulin's major effects include:

* increased glucose transport into adipose tissue, muscle and liver
* increased transmembrane transport of amino acids and increased uptake into muscle
* increased nucleic acid and protein synthesis, and decreased protein catabolism in muscle
* increased glycogen synthesis in muscle and liver
* increased lipogenesis in liver and adipose tissue
* glucose conversion to triglycerides
* promotion of potassium and phosphate entry into cells.

1.25   B: Approximately 95% of the subjects have systolic blood pressures between 101 and 189 mmHg

The distribution of systolic blood pressure is normal or Gaussian, because the mean and median values are equal. Therefore, 95% of observations fall within two standard deviations (not standard errors) of the mean or between 101 and 189 mmHg; 2.5% of the subjects will have a systolic blood pressure greater than 189 mmHg. Approximately 68% of the values lie within one standard deviation of the mean, ie between 123 and 167 mmHg, and 99% of the observations fall within 2.6 standard deviations (SD) of the mean.

1.26   C: The statistical significance of the fall in blood glucose may be analysed by a paired Student's *t*-test

A paired *t*-test could be used to compare the means of the blood glucose in patients before and after administration of the new drug. This is a parametric test, which assumes that the data is normally distributed. Non-parametric tests should be used when the data has a skewed distribution or when data is qualitative. Examples of non-parametric tests include the Mann–Whitney *U* test, chi-square test, Kendall's S score and the Wilcoxon rank sum test. Conventionally, a value of $P < 0.05$ is taken to be statistically significant, ie there is less than a 1 in 20 chance that there is no significant difference between the two groups, thus allowing the null hypothesis to be rejected. If the P value $= 0.01$, 1 in 100 studies would be expected to show a significant effect of the drug on blood glucose by chance alone. If $P = 0.05$, there is a 1 in 20 chance that a significant difference in blood glucose would occur by chance alone.

In a double-blind study neither the researcher nor the patient knows which treatment the patient has been randomised to receive. In a single-blind study either the patient or the doctor does not know (usually the patient).

1.27   B: The sensitivity of the screening test is 96%

Screening test result	Disease	Disease-free
Positive	a	b
Negative	c	d

The sensitivity of a screening test is the test's ability to correctly identify those individuals who truly have disease:

$$= \frac{a}{a+c} = \frac{50}{52} \times 100 = 96.15\%$$

The specificity is the test's ability to correctly identify those individuals who do not have disease:

$$= \frac{d}{b+d} = \frac{4939}{4950} \times 100 = 99.8\%$$

The positive predictive value is the proportion of those who test positive who actually have the disease:

$$= \frac{a}{a+b} = \frac{50}{61} \times 100 = 81.97\%$$

The negative predictive value is the proportion of those who test negative who do not have the disease:

$$= \frac{d}{c+d} = \frac{4339}{4941} \times 100 = 99.96\%$$

The sensitivity and specificity are independent of the disease prevalence in the population being tested. The positive and negative predictive values depend on the prevalence of the disease and may vary from population to population.

1.28 B: Cortisol binds to the mineralocorticoid receptor

Thyroid hormone binds to two receptors, the α and β thyroid hormone receptors. These are members of the nuclear receptor family, and are intracellular. Cortisol binds to both the glucocorticoid and mineralocorticoid receptors with high affinity. ACTH receptors are expressed on the adrenal gland and are G protein-coupled. PPAR gamma is essential for adipocyte differentiation, and is the target of the thioridazine group of glitazone drugs. Insulin causes dimerisation of its receptors and then activates tyrosine kinase activity within the receptor.

1.29 B: Graves' disease is associated with myasthenia gravis

Toxic multinodular goitre is unlikely to respond to antithyroid drugs in the long term, and is an indication for surgery or radioiodine. Graves' disease is associated with other autoimmune diseases, including myasthenia gravis. Carbimazole is not contraindicated in pregnancy, but propylthiouracil is usually used as there are anecdotal accounts of aplasia cutis in the offspring of carbimazole-treated mothers. Smoking is a risk factor for development of Graves' ophthalmopathy, and also predicts worsening of the eye disease after radioactive iodine. Radioactive iodine may exacerbate ophthalmic Graves' disease.

1.30 B: Hypoglycaemia

Adrenal insufficiency can cause hypoglycaemia, hypotension, and hypo-natraemia. It does not cause hypokalaemia. Buccal and skin pigmentation may arise due to the action of ACTH. Eosinophilia, and not neutrophilia, is found in adrenal insufficiency.

1.31   A: Amiodarone

Renal failure causes hypogonadism, and so gynaecomastia. Klinefelter's syndrome (47XXY) also causes hypogonadism. Spironolactone increases sex hormone-binding globulin, and so reduces available androgen. As a result, oestrogen acts unopposed on the breast and causes gynaecomastia. Amiodarone affects the thyroid gland, and is not associated with gynaecomastia. Testicular or adrenal cancers can produce oestrogen and so cause gynaecomastia.

1.32   A: 90% of patients respond to long-acting somatostatin analogue treatment

Around 90% of patients will respond to long-acting somatostatin therapy. Microadenomas have a 90% cure rate in experienced surgical centres. Macroadenomas (> 10 mm in diameter) have a lower cure rate of < 40%. Suprasellar extension does not preclude a trans-sphenoidal approach. The local anatomy of the tumour is important, and is the indication (eg decompression of the optic chiasm). Diabetes occurs in > 10% of acromegalic patients. Hyper-cholesterolaemia is not associated with acromegaly, but cardiovascular disease and increased mortality are.

1.33   B: They are made using human B lymphocytes

Monoclonal antibodies are made by fusing a mouse B cell expressing a specific antibody with a mouse myeloma cell line. The myeloma cells give the B cells immortality, and the resulting hybridoma can be grown *in vitro* indefinitely. The antibodies produced can be purified and used in radioimmunoassays to measure hormones, can be used in histology to look for expression of specific proteins, and can be used therapeutically and *in vitro* to activate T lymphocytes.

1.34   C: They cause 'ragged red' fibres in skeletal muscle

The mitochondrial genome is small and circular. It is exclusively inherited from the mother (sperm contain no mitochondria). The genome is vulnerable to mutations, and inheritance of some mutated mitochondrial chromosomes increases the likelihood of developing disease. The tissues characteristically involved are muscle, brain, nerve and pancreatic islet. Encephalopathy, myopathy, diabetes and lactic acidosis are characteristic features.

1.35   E: It results from amplification of triplet repeats within genes

Genetic anticipation results from the amplification of unstable triplet base repeats within the coding region of genes within affected families. As a result, the size of the repeat increases with successive generations and so the age of onset of disease declines. Huntington's disease and fragile X syndrome are both examples. Turner's syndrome cannot be inherited, and is a chromosomal loss disease.

1.36   D: RNA polymerase II gives rise to protein encoding mRNA

Mammalian mRNA is monocistronic (ie each mRNA encodes one protein), in contrast to bacterial mRNA. RNA polymerase II is responsible for transcribing mRNA. Introns are transcribed, and then spliced out of the RNA to give mature mRNA before the mRNA leaves the nucleus. The genetic code is degenerate, and so multiple codons (triplets of nucleotides) encode the same amino acid. Therefore, not all changes in the nucleotide sequence will give rise to changes in the protein sequence. Usually about 1% of cellular RNA is mRNA; the rest is structural.

1.37   A: Activates the NFkB transcription factor

Tumour necrosis factor-α (TNF-α) can bind a p55 and a p75 receptor. The receptors are coupled to death pathways and so can induce apoptosis in susceptible cells. TNF induces activation of NFkB. TNF has been linked with insulin resistance, especially in obesity. TNF is elevated in synovial fluid, and anti-TNF is useful in treating rheumatoid arthritis. TNF induces expression of other pro-inflammatory cytokines, including IL-1, and IL-6.

1.38   D: Progression from predominantly small peripheral joint disease to involve more proximal, larger joints

Rheumatoid arthritis is a multifactorial disease with an important genetic component. Approximately 20% of identical twins will develop the disease. HLA class II antigen DR4 is associated with disease, and the association is stronger with more severe disease (ie seropositivity; > 70% of seropositive patients are DR4 positive). The typical progression is from peripheral small joints to later involvement of the larger joints, but sacroiliac disease is rare.

1.39   D: Patients have a characteristic reduction in circulating CD8+ T lymphocytes

Polymyalgia rheumatica (PMR) is a disorder of middle aged and elderly patients. Disease is rare before age 45, or after age 80. A third of patients are aged < 60 years. The onset is rapid, with full development in a month. Systemic features include weight loss, night sweats, fever, fatigue and malaise and are common. Muscle enzymes and EMG are normal in PMR. Patients respond rapidly to prednisolone, but so do patients with sepsis, osteoarthritis, and rheumatoid arthritis, and so the improvement is not helpful for diagnosis. There is a characteristic loss of CD8+ T cytotoxic/suppressor cells which can persist up to a year after clinical remission.

1.40   E: Over-represented in Whipple's disease

HLA-B27 is a class I HLA, or major histocompatibility complex (MHC) antigen and is expressed on most cells types. It is over-represented in ankylosing spondylitis (90% of patients compared to 8% of normals), Whipple's disease, reactive arthritis, psoriatic arthritis, Reiter's syndrome, and uveitis. It is not over-represented in Crohn's disease, ulcerative colitis, or Behçet's disease. Class II HLA antigens are expressed on antigen-presenting cells, like dendritic cells, and B lymphocytes.

1.41   C: Polyarteritis nodosa (PAN) mainly affects small vessels

PAN typically affects medium-sized arteries, with frequent aneurysm formation. Antibodies to proteinase-3 (also known as cANCA) are exceptionally rare in non-vasculitic disease. Wegener's granulomatosis affects the upper and lower airways, and the small vessels of the kidney. Patients with Churg–Strauss syndrome typically present with asthma and eosinophilia. An environmental agent is suggested by the seasonal change in incidence shown in North America.

1.42   D: High frequencies of disease are seen in women of Chinese ancestry

SLE is commoner in women with African, Chinese, Asian or South American Indian ancestry, compared to North Europeans. Women are affected more frequently than men (9:1), and there is an increased incidence in Klinefelter's syndrome (47XXY). The skin is a target organ in 70% of cases. Around 15% of the normal population have Raynaud's phenomenon; in SLE the incidence is between 20% and 30%. C-reactive protein is not raised in SLE.

1.43   C: Hyaline casts consist of Tamm–Horsfall protein

Hyaline casts are made of Tamm–Horsfall protein, a mucoprotein secreted by the distal convoluted tubule. They are found in normal urine, more so after exercise, during febrile illness, and after loop diuretics. Oxalate crystals are found in normal urine if it is allowed to stand. When present in freshly passed urine, or in large amounts, they indicate a predisposition to stone formation. Cystine crystals indicate cystinuria. Counts of > 10 white cells per ml urine is abnormal, usually indicating urinary tract infection. A few red cells are found in normal urine; > 2000 per ml is probably abnormal.

1.44   A: Aciclovir

The clearance of a drug depends on size and protein binding. Most antibiotics are small and so are dialysed, with the exception of vancomycin, amphotericin, and erythromycin. Protein-bound drugs like warfarin and propranolol are not cleared.

1.45   D: Urine sodium > 20 mmol/l

Pre-renal failure is caused by poor renal perfusion. The kidney retains sodium (hence urine sodium concentrations are low), and excretes urea (hence urine urea concentrations are high compared to plasma). The urine osmolality is high. Associated features of hypovolaemia should be sought, and these include postural hypotension, and decreased pulmonary wedge pressures.

1.46   B: Abdominal pain is a common presenting feature

The inheritance is autosomal dominant. Abdominal pain, spontaneous haematuria, an increase in girth, hypertension, urinary tract infection, renal colic, and renal impairment may all be presenting features of this disease. There is no specific treatment for the condition, which will require renal replacement therapy between ages 30 and 50 in most cases. A third of patients will have a hepatic cyst, and a few pancreatic or splenic cysts. Berry aneurysms in the cerebral circulation may cause haemorrhage in approximately 10% of patients.

1.47   E: The proximal nephron actively secretes hydrogen ions, in contrast to the distal nephron

Under normal circumstances both the proximal and distal tubule actively secrete hydrogen ions into the tubular fluid. These combine with filtered bicarbonate ions to form carbonic acid, which dissociates into water and carbon dioxide. The carbon dioxide is reabsorbed, and used to generate bicarbonate ions, which are returned to the circulation. Approximately 90% of the bicarbonate ions filtered by the glomerulus are recovered in this manner. In distal renal tubular acidosis there is a mild chronic hyperchloraemic metabolic acidosis (normal anion gap), with exacerbations of acidosis. There is failure of the distal tubule to secrete hydrogen ions, and so the urine pH seldom falls below 5.5. About 70% of patients will have nephrocalcinosis or renal calculi, distinguishing the disorder from the other renal tubular acidoses. Proximal tubular acidosis is rare as an isolated defect, and is often found with aminoaciduria, glycosuria, hyperphosphaturia and uricosuria. The condition is usually part of a Fanconi syndrome but may result from poisoning (eg outdated tetracycline).

1.48   D: It is a lentivirus

HIV is a lentivirus (a virus with slow progression). There are two forms, 1 and 2. Both forms cause AIDS, but disease progression is slower with type 2. The two viruses appear to have distinct evolutionary origins. The HIV viruses are retroviruses, with RNA-containing genomes. HIV gains entry to the cell via a chemokine receptor, and results in depletion of CD4 cells. An adverse indicator is elevation of the CD8 cell count.

1.49   B: Pneumococcal otitis media is usually associated with neutrophil leucocytosis

Pneumococcus is a Gram-positive organism. Pneumococcal pneumonia shows a peak in winter, probably due to low humidity, low temperature, and respiratory virus infection. Otitis media due to *Pneumococcus* is usually associated with neutrophilia, which can be helpful in diagnosis. Pneumococcal meningitis is accompanied by a high mortality rate, even with modern treatment. The disease carries a mortality at least five times greater than that of meningococcal meningitis. Sickle cell disease results in hyposplenism, and so predisposes to pneumococcal disease, which can be prevented by antibody prophylaxis.

1.50   D: Herpes meningitis is a relatively benign condition in adults

Herpes simplex consists of two types: 1, which mainly causes orofacial disease; and 2, which mainly causes genital disease. Herpes meningitis is benign, with normal adults recovering in about a week; no specific treatment is needed. Erythema multiforme frequently results from previous herpes infection. Antibody titres are only useful in retrospective diagnosis on the basis of a rising titre in the convalescent phase. The herpes viruses are double-stranded DNA viruses.

1.51   B: Identification of Gram-positive diplococci on lumbar puncture suggests meningococcal meningitis

Meningococci are Gram-negative diplococci. Acute septicaemia is associated with neutrophilia, as is meningitis; leucopenia is rarely found in fulminating cases. The classic early skin lesion is a petechial rash, but as the condition deteriorates more extensive haemorrhagic lesions develop. Rifampicin eradicates nasal carriage of meningococci in 25% at six days, and 19% at two weeks. Transmission is usually by respiratory droplet, though sexual transmission is also reported.

1.52   D: Haematuria

Typhoid should be suspected in travellers with unexplained fever. The rise in temperature shows gradual onset and reaches 39–40 °C, characteristically with little diurnal variation. The most common associated feature is headache. Classically there is constipation, although most patients will experience loose stools at some time also. Features of significant infection, such as myalgia, lassitude, and arthralgia are not specific. Notable features of untreated infection include altered mental state, which gives typhoid its name. Typically this includes mental apathy and can progress to agitated delirium. Nephrotyphoid is rare and so haematuria usually suggests another cause for the fever.

1.53   A: Aortic dissection is a recognised complication

Mutations in Marfan's syndrome are scattered throughout the gene on chromosome 15 that encodes fibrillin, a component of microfibrils in the extracellular matrix. The mutations are most often missense, that is, they result in an amino acid substitution. The gene contains 65 exons. Marfan's syndrome is inherited in an autosomal dominant fashion with variable expression but generally full penetrance. New mutations occur in about 15–30% of cases. Slit lamp examination is required for detection of slight lens dislocation.

1.54   E: Velocardiofacial syndrome

Aneurysms of the aorta are seen in Marfan's syndrome while intracranial berry aneurysms are observed in polycystic kidney disease. Large vessel rupture is a recognised complication of pseudoxanthoma elasticum (usually autosomal recessive) and of type IV Ehlers–Danlos syndrome (autosomal dominant). Type IV (ie vascular) Ehlers–Danlos syndrome results from a type III collagen defect, whereas the classic forms of Ehlers–Danlos syndrome result from a type V collagen abnormality. Pulmonary arteriovenous shunts, and their potential for spontaneous rupture, are a known complication of hereditary haemorrhagic telangiectasia.

1.55   E: There is no increase in the incidence of homosexuality

The incidence is approximately 1 in 1000 newborn males. There is no association with severe learning difficulties, though the range of IQs in affected individuals is shifted down slightly, relative to that of unaffected individuals. Verbal scores are affected most. There is no increase in the incidence of homosexuality. Breast development is present in around 25–30%. Testosterone therapy is believed to help prevent osteoporosis, in addition to increasing libido and physical activity. Testes are generally much smaller than normal and Leydig cell function is reduced. Spermatogenesis is very poor but in some cases fertilisation may be achieved by sperm aspiration or biopsy, followed by intra-cytoplasmic sperm injection (ICSI).

1.56   C: HNPCC *hMLH1*

FGFR3 (the fibroblast growth factor receptor-3 gene) is associated with achondroplasia. *SMN* (survival motor neurone) is the gene responsible for spinal muscular atrophy (SMA). Limb-girdle muscular dystrophy is associated with the genes for sarcoglycans and calpain, while congenital muscular dystrophy is associated with the gene for merosin. Hereditary non-polyposis colon cancer (HNPCC) is usually associated with mutations in either the *hMLH1* or the *hMSH2* gene.

1.57   D: It exists predominantly as a nucleoprotein complex

Only about 3% of nuclear DNA is coding. The coding sequences are interrupted by introns, which are removed during splicing. Hydrogen bonds mediate base-pairing, while the sugar-phosphate 'backbone' of each DNA strand is held together by covalent bonds. DNA in the nucleus is tightly wrapped around proteins called histones, thus forming a nucleoprotein complex.

NEUROLOGY: 'BEST OF FIVE' ANSWERS

2.1 B: Benign intracranial hypertension (BIH)

Despite raised intracranial pressure causing papilloedema, BIH is a condition in which consciousness is clear and there are no focal neurological signs (though 'false localising' signs, such as a sixth nerve palsy may occur). BIH often presents with headache and transient visual obscurations that presage more permanent visual failure. CT is normal, ie there is no hydrocephalus. Classically, BIH occurs in obese young women but can also be associated with pregnancy, the oral contraceptive pill, hypocortisolism, hypoparathyroidism, hyper- and hypo-vitaminosis A, tetracycline therapy and other drugs. Treatment is with weight loss, serial lumbar puncture, acetazolamide and steroids.

2.2 D: Ulnar nerve

The ulnar nerve is derived from C8 and T1 roots, and in the hand innervates the hypothenar muscles, the third and fourth lumbricals, the interossei and adductor pollicis. Sensory supply is to the fifth finger, the ulnar aspect of the fourth finger and the ulnar border of the palm. The ulnar nerve may be damaged by pressure in the axilla, eg from the use of crutches, but is more commonly damaged at the elbow by trauma. Complete ulnar palsy results in a characteristic claw-hand deformity with hyperextension of the fingers at the metacarpophalangeal joints and flexion at the interphalangeal joints, most pronounced on the ulnar aspect of the hand.

2.3 E: Normal

This is a classic history of optic neuritis. In a third of cases, there will be optic disc oedema of variable severity (and which does not correlate with either field deficit or degree of visual acuity loss), but in the majority of cases the disc appearance is normal. Disc haemorrhages are rare, and pallor generally develops over the two months following the episode. An increase in the cup/disc ratio is a feature of glaucoma.

2.4 C: Lumbar puncture

Subarachnoid haemorrhage (SAH) has not been ruled out by the normal CT. CT is abnormal is only 80–90% of proven SAH, so when SAH is suspected a normal CT should be followed by lumbar puncture and examination of the CSF for xanthochromia.

2.5   D: Communicating hydrocephalus

Normal-pressure hydrocephalus classically presents with the triad of dementia, early onset of urinary incontinence and gait disturbance. Patients may not have all these features, but the CT appearance reveals hydrocephalus with an enlarged fourth ventricle but normal or compressed cortical sulci (ie the pattern of communicating hydrocephalus). Papilloedema is not a clinical feature. Many patients improve with ventricular shunting, though CSF flow studies may identify those patients most likely to improve.

2.6   B: Right occipital lobe

Visual field defects are helpful in localising lesions. Defects restricted to one eye are likely to represent lesions to the retina or optic nerve. Bitemporal field deficits indicate a lesion of the optic chiasm. Homonymous field defects indicate pathology posterior to the chiasm. Quadrantanopia most often indicates a lesion in either the optic radiations or occipital cortex. Superior quadrantanopia indicates damage to the temporal optic radiations or inferior bank of the calcarine (primary visual) cortex. Parietal or superior calcarine lesions will, in contrast, produce an inferior quadrantanopia. Hemianopia typically results from damage to both banks of the calcarine cortex, ie a contralateral occipital lesion.

2.7   C: Brown-Séquard syndrome

This question tests knowledge of spinal cord anatomy, specifically the distinction between crossed and uncrossed sensory pathways. In the spinal cord, fibres carrying vibration and joint-position sense ascend ipsilaterally to the cuneate and gracilis nuclei in the brainstem, where they decussate and ultimately project to contralateral primary sensory cortex in the postcentral gyrus. In contrast, pain and temperature fibres ascend contralaterally in the spinothalamic tracts. Thus, cord hemisection (eg Brown-Séquard syndrome, most commonly associated with multiple sclerosis) can lead to ipsilateral loss of proprioception but contralateral loss of pain sensation. Motor function is lost ipsilaterally in cord hemisection due to interruption of descending corticospinal fibres.

2.8   C: Right abducens

The way in which oculomotor mononeuropathies affect diplopia can be predicted with three rules. First, paresis of horizontally acting muscles causes predominantly horizontal diplopia, and of vertical muscles predominantly causes vertical diplopia. Second, the direction in which the separation of the two images is maximal is the direction of action of the weak muscle. Finally, covering the affected eye leads to disappearance of the outer (false) image. In this case, these suggest right lateral rectus palsy.

2.9   D: Sensitivity

The sensitivity of a test for a particular disease refers to how good that test is at correctly identifying people who have that disease. It represents the probability that the test will produce a true positive result when used on an infected population (as compared to a reference or 'gold standard'). A test with high sensitivity will have few false negatives. The specificity of a test, on the other hand, is concerned with how good the test is at correctly identifying people who are well and do not have a disease. A test with high specificity will have few false positives. The positive predictive value of a test is the probability that a person is infected when a positive test result is observed. On the other hand, the negative predictive value of a test is the probability that a person is not infected when a negative test result is observed. Sensitivity and specificity are both measures of the accuracy of a diagnostic test.

2.10   A: Carbamazepine

This history is typical of trigeminal neuralgia. This is a disorder of the fifth cranial (trigeminal) nerve that causes episodes of intense, stabbing, electric shock-like pain in the distribution of the trigeminal nerve (most frequently, in the maxillary and mandibular divisions). Initial treatment is usually with anticonvulsant drugs, though antidepressants may be helpful. If medication is ineffective or not tolerated, neurosurgical procedures may be required.

2.11   C: Posterior inferior cerebellar artery occlusion

This individual has suffered damage to the lateral medulla, resulting in Wallenberg's syndrome. Wallenberg's syndrome comprises vertigo, nausea, vomiting, ipsilateral cerebellar signs, contralateral sensory disturbance on the body, saccadic abnormalities, dysphagia, dysphonia, dysarthria and a Horner's syndrome. The syndrome is most commonly caused by occlusion of the posterior inferior cerebellar artery or one of its branches supplying the lower brainstem.

2.12   C: Intravenous phenytoin 15 mg/kg

This is established status epilepticus and initial treatment with intravenous lorazepam has not worked. It would not be appropriate to give diazepam (lorazepam and diazepam are equally effective in terminating status but have the same mechanism of action) or a lower dose of lorazepam. In this situation, the best drug to give would be an intravenous infusion of phenytoin at a dose of 15–18 mg/kg. Phenobarbital (phenobarbitone) could also be used, but the typical dosage is 10 mg/kg.

2.13   A: Left angular gyrus

This is Gerstmann's syndrome, which has four principal features: writing disability (agraphia or dysgraphia), lack of understanding of calculation or arithmetic (acalculia or dyscalculia), an inability to distinguish right from left, and an inability to identify fingers (finger agnosia). It can be caused by a lesion (eg stroke) in the angular gyrus of the dominant parietal lobe. In a right-handed individual, the left hemisphere is almost always the dominant hemisphere.

2.14   B: Creutzfeldt–Jakob disease (CJD)

Sporadic CJD predominantly affects late-middle-aged individuals with a mean age at death in the late 60s. Memory impairment and cerebellar ataxia are common early features. Subsequently, rapidly progressive dementia, ataxia and myoclonus are common features. The median duration of illness is four months and about 65% of cases die within six months.

2.15   E: No driving for one year

Medical aspects of fitness to drive in the United Kingdom are described in full at *http://www.dvla.gov.uk/at_a_glance/content.htm*. For a single unprovoked seizure, the regulations state that the patient will lose their licence to drive a private motor vehicle (Group 1) for one year, and will require a medical review before restarting driving.

2.16   E: Propranolol

Prophylactic therapy should be considered in migraine when acute therapy alone is failing to control the symptoms, typically when patients experience more than three or four attacks per month. A variety of agents can be tried, but the most common are β-blockers, amytriptiline and other antidepressants, calcium-channel blockers and anticonvulsants.

2.17   A: Common peroneal nerve

The common peroneal nerve is motor to the peronei and anterior tibial muscles, and damage therefore results in paralysis of dorsiflexion (leading to foot drop) and inability to evert the foot. A lesion above the lateral cutaneous branch results in anaesthesia over the anterolateral lower leg and dorsum of the foot.

2.18   C: Anti-Yo antibodies

Paraneoplastic syndromes are immune-mediated syndromes associated with particular cancers. There are several different CNS-associated paraneoplastic syndromes, but the ataxia here suggests paraneoplastic cerebellar degeneration in the absence of any cerebellar metastases. This occurs most frequently in breast and ovarian malignancy and is associated with anti-Yo antibodies. Treatment of the underlying malignancy may prevent progression of symptoms, but frequently does not result in improvement. Anti-Hu antibodies are often seen in subacute sensorimotor neuropathies associated with small-cell lung cancer. Anti-Ro antibodies are seen in Sjogren's syndrome, SLE and other rheumatological syndromes. Acetylcholine receptor antibodies are characteristic of myasthenia gravis. Finally, calcium channel antibodies are seen in Eaton–Lambert myasthenic syndrome.

2.19   D: Optic neuritis

Optic neuritis typically presents with loss of vision, abnormal colour vision and eye pain. The initial attack is unilateral in about 75% of adult patients, and the mean age of onset is in the third decade.

2.20   C: Toxoplasmosis

Toxoplasmosis is the most frequent cause of intracranial mass lesions in AIDS, causing single or multiple brain abscesses. Clinically, the presentation is heterogeneous, ranging from a febrile illness to focal neurological deficits, developing either subacutely or acutely. Small to medium size ring-enhancing lesions with surrounding oedema on CT suggest the diagnosis.

2.21   C: Carbamazepine

This is a description of simple partial seizures, specifically a focal motor seizure. This would be best treated with carbamazepine, although phenytoin would also be a possibility. Levetiracetam and vigabatrin are primarily used for adjunctive treatment of partial seizures; lorazepam is used in the acute treatment of status epilepticus.

2.22   B: Partially treated bacterial meningitis

This is a typical presentation of a partially treated bacterial meningitis. All of the other options should reduce glucose levels.

2.23   A: Shy–Drager syndrome

The combination of parkinsonism (tremor, rigidity and bradykinesia) with symptoms suggestive of autonomic failure suggest multiple system atrophy, also called Shy–Drager syndrome. Other autonomic symptoms may include sweating abnormalities, gastrointestinal disturbance, abnormal Valsalva response, difficulty with urination or sexual function, and loss of the normal beat-to-beat variability in heart rate.

2.24   A: Tensilon® test

The Tensilon® test involves intravenous injection of edrophonium (a drug that inhibits acetylcholinesterase, enhancing the availability of acetylcholine at the neuromuscular junction). In patients with neuromuscular junction problems, this will lead to a short-acting but clinically definite improvement in muscular strength. Surprisingly, the Tensilon® test is not particularly sensitive or specific and serological tests (for acetylcholine receptor antibodies) or single-fibre electromyography demonstrate better sensitivity and specificity. However, of the tests listed, the Tensilon® test will be the best to confirm the diagnosis.

2.25   C: Multiple system atrophy

All of these diagnoses can be associated with extrapyramidal signs. Typically, the triad of rigidity, resting tremor and bradykinesia is associated with Parkinson's disease. Here, the presence of additional autonomic symptoms and signs suggests a 'Parkinson's plus' syndrome. Postural hypotension may occur in patients with Parkinson's disease, but is typically mild and secondary to (levodopa) medication. Multiple system atrophy represents a group of disorders combining parkinsonism with moderate to severe autonomic neuropathy. In this group of disorders, the parkinsonism is typically poorly responsive to treatment.

2.26   C: Right abducens nerve

Three cranial nerves control the upper eyelid, eye movements and pupils, the oculomotor (third), trochlear (fourth) and abducens (sixth). Horizontal diplopia implies a weakness of the horizontally acting muscles, vertical diplopia the vertically acting muscles. Diplopia is maximal in the direction of action of the weak muscle, and when the eye to which the weak muscle belongs is covered, then the outer (false) image is obscured. Thus, in this case, the diplopia is caused by a weak right lateral rectus, thus indicating right abducens palsy. This is most likely to have been caused by poorly controlled diabetes mellitus.

2.27   E: Temporal lobe uncus across the tentorium

Space-occupying lesions can impair consciousness either through direct extension of the lesion into the midbrain and brainstem or, more commonly, by lateral and downward displacement of these structures with or without herniation of the medial part of the temporal lobe through the tentorium. This lateral displacement typically crushes the upper midbrain against the opposite free edge of the tentorium, causing an upgoing plantar ipsilateral to the hemispheric lesions. All forms of brainstem herniation can cause depression of respiration, extensor posturing and bilateral upgoing plantars. The uncal syndrome differs mainly in that early drowsiness is accompanied or preceded by unilateral pupillary dilatation, often (but not always) due to compression of the oculomotor nerve by the herniated uncus.

2.28   C: Posterior inferior cerebellar artery

Ipsilateral Horner's syndrome and contralateral loss of pain and temperature sensation indicate damage in the dorsolateral region of the medulla, known as Wallenberg's syndrome. Lower vestibular nuclei are often involved, resulting in vertigo, vomiting and nystagmus; involvement of the inferior cerebellar peduncle will result in ipsilateral limb ataxia. This medullary syndrome is most often caused by occlusion of the posterior inferior cerebellar artery, although in some cases an occlusion of the parent vertebral artery can be responsible.

2.29   A: Acoustic neuroma

A cerebellopontine angle lesion is indicated by the combination of absent corneal reflex and sensorineural deafness. No other single central lesion could account for these signs. Lesions arising in the pons, such as multiple sclerosis or brainstem astrocytoma, are likely to present with more complex neurological signs. Similarly, extrinsic lesions, such as basilar artery aneurysm or nasopharyngeal carcinoma, are more likely to present with isolated single compressive cranial nerve lesions.

2.30   C: Left thalamic metastasis

The dense sensory impairment described here is typical for a space-occupying thalamic lesion and the progressive history over several months makes metastasis more likely than either demyelination or stroke. Sensory loss caused by a cortical lesion is rarely complete.

2.31   A: Craniopharyngioma

Craniopharyngiomas compress the optic chiasm from above and behind, producing a bitemporal hemianopia that spreads up from the lower fields into the upper fields. In adults, pituitary dysfunction secondary to craniopharyngioma is variable, but the tumour may block the third ventricle causing hydrocephalus and dementia. Pituitary macroadenomas cause a bitemporal hemianopia which typically spreads down from the upper fields as the optic chiasm is damaged from below.

2.32   A: Common peroneal nerve

The common peroneal nerve is most often damaged by compression at the fibula neck, where it winds around the bone. The nerve is motor to tibialis anterior and the peronei, causing weakness of dorsiflexion and eversion respectively. As nerve roots L5 and S1 control these movements, differentiation from an L5 root lesion requires demonstration of intact eversion in the presence of severe weakness of dorsiflexion. The common peroneal nerve is sensory to a small patch of skin on the dorsum of the foot between the big and second toes, but often there is little or no sensory loss detectable clinically.

2.33   C: Meningococcal meningitis

This patient has an acute bacterial meningitis, and is predisposed to infection due to his splenectomy. Meningococcal meningitis is the most likely diagnosis, due to the characteristic petechiae and purpura. Although these skin manifestations can also be seen occasionally with *Haemophilus* and pneumococcal meningitis, they are much more common in meningococcal meningitis.

2.34   D: Episodic memory deficit

The gradual development of forgetfulness is the major symptom of Alzheimer's disease, and is characterised on neuropsychological testing by a deficit of episodic memory. Other failures of cortical function, including all the disorders here, may be manifest but typically occur later in the course of the disease. Visual hallucinations are often a prominent feature of a less common form of dementia, corticobasal degeneration; and frontal syndromes, such as disinhibition, together with progressive language impairment, are seen in Pick's disease.

2.35   A: Huntington's disease

Progressive chorea, emotional disturbance and dementia with onset in the fourth decade are typical of Huntington's disease. Patients may lack or conceal a family history; diagnosis is usually easy, as the mutation (CAG repeat expansion in the Huntington gene) has been identified. The other diagnoses listed here can cause an extrapyramidal movement disorder, but choreiform movements are less common and/or prominent, and intellectual decline is not typically a presenting feature.

2.36   C: Left parietal lobe

This woman has a partial Gerstmann's syndrome, affecting the dominant (left) parietal lobe. The characteristic features are inability to name the fingers of the two hands (finger agnosia), confusion of left and right sides of the body, inability to calculate (dyscalculia) or write (dysgraphia). Damage to the superior part of the optic radiation in the underlying white matter causes a contralateral homonymous lower quadrantanopia (in contrast to the homonymous superior quadrantanopia following temporal lesions). Often the patient will be unaware of the visual field deficit.

2.37   D: Haeme

Severe symmetric polyneuropathy, together with abdominal pain and neuro-psychiatric symptoms (or confusion), is typical of acute intermittent porphyria. This is a disorder of haem metabolism inherited as an autosomal dominant syndrome, with attacks often precipitated by drugs such as oestrogens, phenytoin and sulphonamides. The neuropathy often involves the motor nerves more severely than the sensory; symptoms may begin in the arms or legs, usually distally but occasionally also in the proximal limb girdle.

2.38   B: Guillain–Barré syndrome

Guillain–Barré syndrome (GBS) is an acute ascending polyneuropathy; as here, sensory symptoms are typically out of proportion to the weakness. Areflexia is characteristic and progression can be rapid with respiratory failure and death. The most immediate diagnostic problem is to differentiate GBS from acute spinal cord compression (which would produce an upper motor neurone lesion in the legs with hyper-reflexia and upgoing plantars, and does not produce facial weakness). CSF is typically acellular or shows a mild lymphocytosis, but with a grossly elevated protein.

2.39   A: Carbamazepine

This woman has complex partial seizures, with a typical aura followed by loss of consciousness and subsequent post-ictal confusion. While unconscious during the fit, her behaviour shows automatisms and semipurposive features. Carbamazepine is the drug of choice for complex partial seizures, or sometimes sodium valproate. Phenytoin can be successful but can also sometimes worsen complex partial seizures. Lamotrigine, vigabatrin and gabapentin are also useful, but only as second-line agents.

2.40   E: Sagittal sinus

Parasagittal biparietal or bifrontal haemorrhagic infarctions are common sequelae of sagittal sinus thrombosis. Oral contraceptives, the immediate post-partum period, hypercoagulable states and dehydration all predispose to sagittal sinus thrombosis. The presence of multiple lesions which are not in typical arterial territories, and the prominent epileptic fits, favour this diagnosis.

2.41   E: Vitamin B$_{12}$

Subacute combined degeneration of the spinal cord, due to vitamin B$_{12}$ deficiency, results in degeneration of the posterior columns (vibration and joint-position sense), followed by progressive development of upper motor neurone signs in the legs. Spinal cord involvement is roughly symmetrical, but can progress to dementia and visual impairment due to optic neuropathy. Thiamine deficiency may give rise to Wernicke's syndrome (ophthalmoplegia, ataxia and confusion), or to beri-beri (peripheral neuropathy). Pyridoxine deficiency gives rise to a chronic painful sensorimotor neuropathy. This can be caused by administration of isoniazid (for tuberculosis), which increases the excretion of pyridoxine; hence isoniazid is always administered in conjunction with pyridoxine.

2.42   D: Radial

The radial nerve in the axilla is often damaged by the incorrect use of a crutch, which causes weakness of all the radial nerve-innervated muscles. In addition to triceps and the wrist and finger extensors, there is also weakness of brachioradialis. Triceps is only variably involved, for reasons that are unclear.

2.43   B: Creutzfeldt–Jakob disease

This is a rapidly progressive and severe dementia associated with cerebellar ataxia, diffuse myoclonic jerks, and other neurological abnormalities. Myoclonus is typical and progressive, even during the later stages when the patient is stuporous or comatose. The disease is invariably fatal, usually within a few months. The EEG pattern is characteristic but diagnosis relies on either specialised tests for prion protein in CSF, or direct brain biopsy.

2.44   C: Dextroamphetamine

This individual has narcolepsy (the sudden irresistible urge to sleep) and cataplexy (sudden loss of muscle tone following strong emotions or excitement). Cataplexy is seen in up to 70% of patients with narcolepsy, either at diagnosis or later in the disease. In narcolepsy, rapid eye movement (REM) sleep occurs within 15 minutes in most subjects. Sleepiness is the main problem here, so treatment with stimulant drugs (amphetamine) to heighten alertness is most appropriate; however, imipramine may also be useful for cataplexy.

PSYCHIATRY: 'BEST OF FIVE' ANSWERS

3.1   E: Cerebral involvement is an indicator of poor prognosis

CNS involvement occurs in about a third of cases of SLE. Psychiatric symptoms occur in 60% of cases: the excess is due to both psychological reactions to illness and corticosteroid side-effects. The most common presentations are acute organic states and neurotic disorders; schizophrenia-like syndromes are rare. Mental symptoms are seldom the first signs of SLE (which are usually fever, malaise and arthralgia). When present, psychiatric symptoms often fluctuate, usually remit within six weeks, but may recur. The presence of cerebral vasculitis substantially worsens prognosis.

3.2   D: It is associated with reduced life expectancy in severe schizophrenia

Tardive dyskinesia is characterised by chewing, sucking and grimacing of the face and choreoathetoid movements. It occurs in about one fifth of patients receiving long-term treatment with neuroleptic medication such as phenothiazines or butyrophenones. Increased incidence is seen in women and with increasing age but not with brain damage or previous treatment with ECT. Few treatments are helpful and stopping the offending drug may produce paradoxical worsening. There is decreased life expectancy when functional psychosis and severe dyskinesia are both present.

3.3   C: Clouding of consciousness

Puerperal psychosis is not thought to be a distinct form of mental illness. It has a number of features in common with post-operative psychoses, including acute confusion and therefore clouding of consciousness. The disorder can present with features similar to an affective or schizophreniform psychosis. Clinical features may therefore include labile mood, overactivity, hallucinations and delusions. Onset is most commonly between two and fourteen days after parturition. A past history of mental illness may be present, but making a diagnosis depends more on the presence of active symptoms at the time of assessment.

3.4   A: A clear history of blackouts with cognitive deficits on assessment

The alcohol dependence syndrome has seven key characteristics. These include a compulsion to drink, withdrawal symptoms, drinking to avoid withdrawal symptoms, altered tolerance, primacy of drink-seeking behaviour over other activities, a stereotyped pattern of drinking and reinstatement of drinking pattern after a period of abstinence, (eg during an inpatient stay). Cognitive deficits and a history of blackouts (inability to recall events which occurred during a period of drinking) can occur in alcohol dependency but are not necessary for the diagnosis.

3.5   B: ECT can cause short-term memory loss

Randomised controlled trials have compared ECT to 'sham' ECT (the application of a general anaesthetic and muscle relaxant but no subsequent ECT). ECT is superior to sham ECT in the treatment of severe depression. Antidepressants are also useful in the treatment of severe depression, but ECT produces quicker results. Therefore, in potentially life-threatening situations, ECT is the treatment of choice. ECT results in brief memory disturbances after each treatment. There is less conclusive evidence that it causes any long-term cognitive impairment. As muscle relaxants are used, patients do not convulse in an uncontrolled manner.

3.6   C: Improvement of mood every evening

Antidepressants are most effective when a patient has evidence of clinical depression. Clinical features include: persistent depressed mood accompanied by guilt or worthlessness; persistent low levels of concentration, energy, appetite and libido; early-morning wakening and diurnal variation of mood, with depression being consistently worse in the morning. The presence of these symptoms suggests an underlying chemical imbalance which can respond to antidepressants.

3.7   B: There is an accompanying sense of impending doom

Panic disorder consists of unpredictable attacks of severe anxiety. Attacks include somatic and psychological symptoms. The latter include a fear that something drastic is about to happen, such as collapse or death. As a consequence, patients often try to hurriedly escape the situation they are in. The attacks last between a few minutes and half an hour and are rarely longer in duration. Continuous feelings of nervousness are more typical of generalised anxiety disorder.

3.8   A: Abnormal psychomotor activity

Delirium is an acute-onset syndrome characterised by inattention and an impaired level of consciousness. Thinking is often disorganised and perseverative. Perceptual disturbances include misinterpretations, illusions and hallucinations. There is disturbance of the sleep-wake cycle, with insomnia and daytime sleepiness. Psychomotor activity may be increased or decreased. Disorientation and memory impairment are common. The patient has no insight during episodes of confusion and amnesia for the episode once it has resolved. 'Catastrophic reaction' has been described in dementing patients, which is characterised by marked agitation secondary to the subjective awareness of intellectual deficits under stressful circumstances.

3.9   D: Olanzapine

Carbamazepine and lithium are both mood stabilisers. Although they can help with symptoms of hypomania, they have more of a role in prophylaxis, to prevent future episodes. More rapid symptom improvement is obtained from antipsychotics such as olanzapine or from benzodiazepines. ECT also produces a rapid response, but would not be indicated as first-line treatment.

3.10   C: Hallucinations in clear consciousness

Abnormal liver function tests, the diagnosis of alcohol dependence syndrome or the presence of insomnia may not help distinguish between alcoholic hallucinosis and delirium tremens. Hallucinations may occur in delirium tremens and are primarily visual. As the name delirium tremens suggests, hallucinations are often accompanied by a clouding of consciousness. In alcoholic hallucinosis, auditory hallucinations are heard in clear consciousness.

3.11   E: Suicidal intent

Alcohol dependence and schizophrenia are both associated with a 10% risk of eventual suicide. When performing a risk assessment one would ask whether the patient no longer feels life is worth living. If so, have they entertained any thoughts about suicide? If so, do they have a plan to kill themselves? A direct statement of intention to commit suicide would be most concerning and should prompt urgent psychiatric referral.

3.12   B: A denial that she is underweight

Anorexia nervosa is characterised by deliberate self-induced weight loss. Key features include body image distortion, with underweight patients believing they are fat. As a consequence of self-induced weight loss, there are endocrine abnormalities which result in amenorrhoea. Her BMI is less than 17.5 kg/m^2, the lower limit for post-pubertal women. However, the BMI is less important as a diagnostic factor than the abnormal psychopathology described above.

3.13   A: Chlordiazepoxide

Clozapine and haloperidol are antipsychotics. Procyclidine is an anticholinergic drug which is often prescribed to individuals who develop extrapyramidal side-effects from antipsychotics. Sodium valproate is prescribed less often, but has been indicated for individuals with prominent affective components to their schizophrenic illness. Chlordiazepoxide is a benzodiazepine used in alcohol detoxification.

3.14   A: Anorgasmia

SSRIs are effective antidepressants with a less sedative effect than tricyclics, few antimuscarinic effects and low carditoxicity. The most frequent side-effects are gastrointestinal (diarrhoea, nausea and vomiting), which are dose-related. Restlessness, anxiety, insomnia and sweating may be marked initially. Side-effects also include anorexia, weight loss and allergic reactions, including anaphylaxis (all more common with fluoxetine), convulsions (particularly with fluvoxamine), extrapyramidal reactions and a withdrawal syndrome (particularly with paroxetine), abnormalities of hepatic enzymes (particularly with fluvoxamine and sertraline) and sexual dysfunction, including anorgasmia and ejaculatory failure in males (particularly with paroxetine and fluoxetine). Suicidal ideation has been associated with SSRIs but causality has not been established.

3.15   D: Reduced volume of the third ventricle

Studies report a significant increase in average lateral ventricle size in schizophrenics compared with normal controls, although with a marked overlap between the two populations. Third ventricle and cortical sulcal enlargement has also been reported. Medial temporal lobe structures appear reduced in volume, particularly on the left, and MRI has revealed widespread grey matter (but not white matter) on the volume deficits.

3.16   D: Low voltage with triphasic discharges

The EEG in CJD initially shows diffuse or focal slowing which is non-specific to this disorder. Later, repetitive sharp waves or slow spike-and-wave discharges appear, which are bilaterally synchronous and may accompany myoclonic jerks. In the later stages of the disorder a characteristic pattern emerges of synchronous triphasic sharp-wave complexes, superimposed on progressive suppression of cortical background activity. The sharp-wave complexes become increasingly periodic at rates of one to two per second. Four-per-second spike-and-wave discharges occur in juvenile absence seizures. Frontal intermittent rhythmic delta activity occurs in metabolic encephalopathy and in brainstem dysfunction.

3.17   B: Caudate atrophy

The patient may not be aware of a family history for a number of reasons, including estrangement from family or intellectual deterioration. Huntington's disease is an uncommon autosomal dominant disorder affecting four to seven people per 100 000 of the population. Senile and drug-induced choreas are much more frequently encountered. Anatomically, the frontal lobes and the caudate nucleus are most severely affected by neuronal loss and gliosis. Ventricular dilatation does occur in Huntington's disease but is less specific than the finding of caudate atrophy.

3.18   A: Alzheimer's dementia

Individuals with mental retardation are at a higher risk of developing a number of mental illnesses, such as schizophrenia or a mood disorder. Epilepsy is found in over 10% of those with Down's syndrome aged over 40. Alzheimer's dementia is found in approximately 95% of individuals with Down's syndrome aged over 40.

3.19   C: Quetiapine

Typical antipsychotics all have some D2 antagonist activity and can thus produce parkinsonian side-effects. Sulpiride acts exclusively on D2 receptors. Haloperidol acts at a number of receptor sites, but is a potent D2 antagonist. Chlorpromazine acts as a weaker D2 antagonist. All atypical antipsychotics have a much lower propensity to produce parkinsonian side-effects. However, at high doses risperidone can produce extrapyramidal side-effects.

3.20   A: Autochthonous delusions

Psychosis is defined as the presence of delusions, hallucinations or specific abnormalities of behaviour, such as catatonia, severe psychomotor retardation or overactivity. Autochthonous (primary) delusions are first-rank symptoms of schizophrenia. Hallucinations of any modality are a feature of psychosis. Hypnagogic and hypnapompic hallucinations are exceptions as they refer to auditory hallucinations experienced not in clear consciousness, but respectively as one drifts into sleep or awakens. Echopraxia is a feature of cognitive impairment. Tardive dyskinesia may be a result of long-term antipsychotic medication, but does not indicate current psychosis.

3.21   B: Catalepsy

Catatonia is a disorder of motor activity and can occur in schizophrenia. Catalepsy, also known as 'waxy' flexibility, is a disorder of muscle tone, which can result in patients maintaining what are often very uncomfortable postures for long periods of time without moving. Stupor, excitement and negativism are other features of catatonia. Cataplexy is the sudden loss of muscle tone. Stereotypes are repeated non-goal-directed movements, eg rocking to and fro. Mannerisms are goal-directed movements that occur out of context.

3.22   C: Prognathism

Fragile X syndrome is the second commonest cause of mental retardation in males. Clinical features include macro-orchidism and facial abnormalities, such as prognathism and hypertelorism. A single palmar crease can occur in fragile X but also occurs in Down's syndrome. Strabismus occurs more frequently with Down's syndrome. Learning difficulties accompanied by an absence of male secondary sexual characteristics is associated with Klinefelter's syndrome. Tall stature is more commonly associated with XYY sex chromosome abnormalities.

3.23   A: A nephew has been diagnosed with schizophrenia

There are several well-documented risk factors for schizophrenia. The most important risk factor is genetic, with increased risk associated with an affected first- or second-degree relative. A history of a winter birth is more common in schizophrenia and may be related to maternal viral infection during pregnancy. Being Afro-Caribbean in itself is not related to increased risk of schizophrenia, but Afro-Caribbean migrants to the UK do show an increase in incidence of schizophrenia. Children who subsequently develop schizophrenia are more likely to have a history of developmental delay and behavioural and interpersonal difficulties. There is equal gender incidence of schizophrenia, although males often present earlier.

3.24   C: The presence of secondary gain

Munchausen's syndrome is a factitious disorder. This disorder is defined as the voluntary production of physical or psychological symptoms, which can be attributed to a need to adopt the sick role. Secondary gain is defined as the presence of an advantage gained as a result of having symptoms – in this case attention and admission. Munchausen's syndrome specifically differs from malingering in that there is no fraudulent simulation of symptoms. Financial gain is therefore not a motive. Alcohol dependence may be present but is not particularly associated with the syndrome. Simulated psychiatric symptoms are common, such as 'hearing voices'. Hearing voices inside one's head is a pseudohallucination and therefore not a true psychotic phenomenon. Voices heard outside one's head is more characteristic of a genuine hallucination.

3.25   E: Bradycardia

Neuroleptic malignant syndrome is a rare but potentially life-threatening complication of neuroleptic therapy. It consists of mental state changes, including confusion and mutism, as well as physical abnormalities. Autonomic dysfunction, including elevated or labile blood pressure, tachycardia, pyrexia and diaphoresis can occur, as well as dysphagia, tremor and incontinence. Treatment varies, depending on the severity of presentation, but always includes the cessation of antipsychotic therapy.

3.26   D: Lofexidine

Lofexidine is the drug of choice for treating opiate withdrawal. It is a central α_2 agonist and helps alleviate the symptoms of opiate withdrawal. A reducing regime of methadone can also be used to help withdraw from opiates. Diamorphine for the treatment of addiction can only be prescribed by doctors specifically licensed to prescribe to addicts. Benzodiazepines and neuroleptics can help relieve symptoms, but are not as effective as lofexidine. Bupropion is a noradrenaline (norepinephrine) and dopamine re-uptake inhibitor and is prescribed as an aid to smoking cessation.

3.27   C: Primary delusion

All of the options listed are features of schizophrenia. A delusion is a false, unshakeable belief out of keeping with a patient's social and cultural background. Primary delusions appear suddenly and with full conviction. Delusional perceptions are examples of primary delusions and are of first-rank importance in the diagnosis of schizophrenia. A delusional perception occurs when an individual forms an instantaneous delusion after a normal perception, for example suddenly believing you are Jesus on seeing a blue car drive past. A secondary delusion is derived from an abnormal mental phenomenon, for example believing oneself to be Jesus because the hallucinatory voice of God has told you so. Other first-rank symptoms are audible thoughts, third-person auditory hallucinations, passivity, and thought broadcasting, insertion or withdrawal.

3.28   E: Self-induced vomiting

The most important feature of anorexia nervosa is that low weight is self-induced. This may be by the restriction of 'fattening foods' from the diet, self-induced vomiting or purging, excessive exercising or the use of appetite suppressants or diuretics. Body image is distorted, with sufferers not accepting that they are underweight. There is also a widespread endocrine disturbance producing a number of symptoms, including amenorrhoea in women. Appetite is usually present but consciously suppressed. The BMI is calculated by dividing weight in kg by height in metres squared (kg/m^2) and in anorexia is 17.5 or less. Lower BMIs could also result from starvation from other causes.

3.29   A: Cognitive behavioural therapy

The patient described has features of clinical depression. Key diagnostic features are depressed mood, increased fatiguability and anhedonia (loss of interest and enjoyment). Trials of different kinds of psychotherapy are difficult to conduct. However, for cases of mild to moderate depression, cognitive behavioural therapy (CBT) has been shown to be as effective as antidepressants.

3.30   A: Anxiety in crowded places

Agoraphobia is defined as a fear of the related aspects of open spaces. This would include the presence of crowds and difficulty escaping to a safe place – usually home. This fear characteristically leads to avoidance of the phobic situation, hence a possible reason for poor attendance in clinic. Anxiety and panic attacks in agoraphobia are predictable and linked to the phobic situation. Unpredictable panic attacks are part of panic disorder. Anxiety predominant in social situations occurs in social phobia.

3.31   E: Thought alienation

Thought alienation is a disorder of the possession of thought. The individual has the experience that his thoughts are under the control of an outside person or force. Examples of thought alienation include thought withdrawal, thought insertion and thought broadcasting. Hallucinations are perceptions experienced without any external stimulus. Hallucinations heard when going to sleep (hypnagogic) or on waking (hypnapompic) can occur in tired, healthy people and in sleep disorders such as narcolepsy. Depersonalisation occurs when a person feels numb and unreal. Derealisation occurs when his environment feels unreal. Both states are unpleasant and occur in a large number of psychiatric disorders, especially anxiety states, depression and schizophrenia. They can also occur in tired, healthy individuals.

3.32   A: Amphetamine

Amphetamines can produce a schizophrenia-like illness in otherwise healthy individuals. Cannabis is thought to bring on schizophrenia early in susceptible individuals, but is otherwise unlikely to produce a schizophreniform psychosis. LSD and psilocybin (found in magic mushrooms) produce perceptual abnormalities, mainly during intoxication, but do not produce first-rank schizophrenic symptoms. Heroin use does not produce psychotic symptoms.

3.33   A: Inability to feel sadness

Uncomplicated grief reactions consist of three stages. The first stage should only last a maximum of a few days and is characterised by denial and numbness. The second stage can last up to six months or one year. This stage is characterised by intense sadness, loneliness, yearning for the dead person, anorexia, poor sleep and anxiety. Fleeting hallucinations of the dead person may also occur. In the third stage symptoms subside and there is gradual acceptance and readjustment. Pathological grief consists of a delayed, inhibited or abnormally long period of grieving. There may also be a typical depressive picture with marked feelings of worthlessness, psychomotor retardation or functional impairment.

3.34   D: Intrusive flashbacks

Repeated reliving of trauma through flashbacks (intrusive memories) or nightmares is typical, with avoidance of situations that might trigger painful memories. The traumatic event must be exceptionally violent or catastrophic in nature. There is often accompanying autonomic hyperarousal, emotional blunting, anhedonia and other features of anxiety and depression, but these are not essential to make the diagnosis. Believing his attackers have followed him to the UK is suggestive of a persecutory delusion, which is not typical of PTSD.

3.35   A: Global memory loss

Patients with depressive pseudodementia are often detailed historians, but perform badly on tests of cognitive functioning. Patients with dementia often demonstrate recent memory loss, whereas those with depression complain of global memory loss. Both groups may have poor concentration, but patients with dementia often make more of an effort with testing. Parietal lobe abnormalities such as dyspraxias or topographical disorientation should not occur in depression.

3.36   E: Somatisation disorder

Somatisation disorder is characterised by multiple, changing physical symptoms that have been present for at least two years. As a result of the symptoms, the patient's life becomes considerably disrupted. However, the patient refuses to accept reassurance from negative test results and medical opinion. In hypochondriacal disorder the patient's focus is not on the symptoms, but on the presence of an underlying serious disease such as cancer or cardiovascular disease. The terms dissociative (psychiatric) and conversion (physical) disorder have replaced the old-fashioned and imprecise term, 'hysteria'.

3.37   B: Intellectual deterioration

Approximately 60% of sufferers with multiple sclerosis demonstrate a degree of intellectual deterioration. This can vary from mild memory loss to profound global dementia. Fleeting mood disorders are very common, with major depressive episodes occurring in approximately half of sufferers. Euphoria occurs in about 10% and is commonly associated with severe cognitive impairment. Psychotic episodes are rare.

3.38   D: Korsakoff's syndrome

Hyperemesis can result in acute thiamine deficiency and subsequent Wernicke's encephalopathy. The majority of cases then progress to Korsakoff's psychosis, a type of amnesic syndrome. Characteristic features of amnesic syndrome include temporal disorientation and very poor retention of recent memories. This is tested by immediate and five-minute recall. Registration of new information will be intact, but recall several minutes later will be impaired. Confabulation can also occur, where detailed memories are recalled which turn out to be inaccurate.

3.39   E: Negativism

Schizophrenic symptoms can be divided into positive and negative. Positive symptoms often occur in acute episodes and include hallucinations, delusions, formal thought disorder and bizarre behaviour. Negative symptoms are associated with a more chronic picture and may be very disabling. These symptoms include poverty of speech (alogia), poor motivation and initiative (avolition), an inability to derive pleasure from activities (anhedonia), emotional blunting and attentional deficits. Catatonia can occur in schizophrenia and is a disorder of psychomotor activity. Symptoms include stupor, excitement, waxy flexibility, mutism and negativism.

3.40   C: Perseverating responses

Frontal lobe dysfunction can result in personality changes, disinhibition and euphoria, or apathy and slowing of thought and motor activity. Perseveration of actions and difficulties in planning and executing actions can also occur. Impaired five-minute recall can suggest bilateral temporal lobe dysfunction. Sensory dysphasia can occur if the dominant temporal lobe is affected. Right-left disorientation is part of Gerstmann's syndrome, affecting the dominant parietal lobe. Hypersomnia may result from dysfunction of the diencephalon and brainstem.

3.41   B: Obsessive-compulsive disorder

A number of psychiatric and physical illnesses are associated with increased risk of suicide. Despite high rates of morbidity and considerably impaired functioning, the suicide rate in obsessive-compulsive disorder (OCD) is considerably lower than in depressed patients without OCD.

3.42   D: Intramuscular lorazepam

In a patient who is neuroleptic-naïve, antipsychotics should be administered with caution. Parenteral administration should be avoided if possible until the response to an oral dose has been assessed. Reasons include an increased risk of cardiovascular complications when antipsychotics are administered parenterally to highly agitated individuals. There is also the risk of acute dystonic reactions. Chlorpromazine, in addition, is highly irritant when administered intramuscularly. Benzodiazepines, often followed by oral antipsychotics, are generally a safer option in this situation. Intramuscular diazepam, however, is poorly absorbed.

3.43   C: Fluctuating recall

Dissociative disorders are examples of 'psychogenic' disorders which do not have sufficient evidence of a physical disorder to explain the symptoms. In dissociative amnesia there is a persistent core of amnesia, which cannot be recalled. However the extent and completeness of amnesia varies from day to day and between investigators. The accompanying affect can vary from distress with attention-seeking to calm acceptance. Disorientation or disturbances of consciousness or awareness would indicate an organic disorder.

3.44   B: Sentences spoken are connected by clanging

Thought disorder occurs when there is a loss of the normal, logical progression of thinking. There are a number of types of schizophrenic thought disorder, including derailment (A), incoherence (B) and illogicality. In mania, thought disorder can occur in the form of flight of ideas. Thoughts follow each other rapidly, with the connection between them often based on verbal associations, such as rhyming, alliteration or clanging, eg 'My car is a rover. Rover is a great dog. Fancy a snog?'

3.45   A: Acknowledging that this belief is irrational, but still refusing

Obsessional thoughts often involve contamination as a theme. They may involve an accompanying compulsive act or ritual that lessens the anxiety associated with the thought. The ritual itself is not inherently pleasurable. Obsessional thoughts must be recognised as the individual's own thoughts and are therefore not part of a psychotic process. The thoughts are commonly perceived as being senseless and are resisted, but at a cost of considerable anxiety.

3.46   E: Short-term memory loss

All of the sequelae listed can occur after a head injury. However, short-term memory loss is usually the most persistent cognitive dysfunction. Focal brain pathology after a head injury can result in focal deficits. For example, executive dysfunction, including impaired planning and executing of actions, can occur with frontal lobe pathology.

3.47   A: Ataxia

The answer to this question is ataxia as you have been asked which abnormality is most likely to indicate toxicity. Tremor can occur at therapeutic plasma levels, whereas ataxia should only occur in toxicity. Lithium has a low therapeutic index, but can produce a number of unpleasant side-effects at therapeutic levels (0.4–1.1 mmol/l). These include fine tremor, nausea, vomiting, diarrhoea and metallic taste. A coarse tremor, ataxia, slurred speech, disorientation and convulsions can occur in toxicity.

3.48   C: Fasciculations

Conversion disorders frequently present to doctors. They are characterised by the presence of symptoms or deficits involving voluntary motor or sensory functions. In motor conversion disorders, the patient may not be able to contract a particular muscle group. However, tests often show that the muscles are able to contract when the patient's attention is diverted. Changes in reflexes are not present, but disuse atrophy can occur in chronic cases.

3.49   E: The majority of cases are preceded by anorexia nervosa

To make a diagnosis of bulimia nervosa there must be recurrent episodes of binge eating – eating larger than normal amounts of food, accompanied by a loss of control over eating. In addition there must be recurrent compensatory behaviour to prevent weight gain, eg self-induced vomiting, laxative or diuretic abuse, fasting or excessive exercising. A fear of fatness is also prominent. About a third of patients with bulimia may previously have had anorexia nervosa. If all features are present apart from compensatory behaviour, the condition is known as binge-eating disorder.

3.50   E: Hallucinations must occur in clear consciousness

Alcoholic hallucinosis is characterised by second-person auditory hallucinations of a derogatory or persecutory nature. Hallucinations occur in clear consciousness and are therefore not part of a delirium or other acute withdrawal syndrome. Hallucinations lasting for more than six months generally develop into either a schizophrenic or an amnesic syndrome.

REVISION CHECKLISTS

BASIC SCIENCES: REVISION CHECKLIST

Physiology

- [ ] Changes in pregnancy
- [ ] Haemoglobin function
- [ ] Physiology of bone
- [ ] Aetiology of oedema
- [ ] Magnesium
- [ ] Exercise

Pathology

- [ ] Amyloid plaques

Hormone and mediator biochemistry

- [ ] Atrial natriuretic peptides
- [ ] Insulin/insulin resistance
- [ ] Adenosine
- [ ] ADH
- [ ] Aldosterone
- [ ] Angiotensin
- [ ] EDRF (nitric oxide)
- [ ] H_2 receptors
- [ ] Neurotransmitters
- [ ] Prostacyclin
- [ ] Somatostatin
- [ ] Steroid receptors

Miscellaneous

- [ ] Apolipoproteins
- [ ] Alpha$_1$-antitrypsin
- [ ] Mitochondrial DNA function
- [ ] Oncogenes
- [ ] Statistics
- [ ] Anatomy
- [ ] Genetics

NEUROLOGY: REVISION CHECKLIST

Abnormalities of brain & cerebral circulation

- [ ] Dementia/Alzheimer's
- [ ] Transient ischaemic attacks
- [ ] Benign intracranial hypertension/brain tumour
- [ ] Head injury
- [ ] Lateral medullary/circulatory syndromes
- [ ] Subdural haematoma
- [ ] Encephalitis
- [ ] Parietal lobe/frontal cortical lesions
- [ ] Temporal lobe epilepsy
- [ ] Amnesia
- [ ] Central pontine myelinolysis
- [ ] Cerebral abscess
- [ ] Creutzfeldt-Jakob disease
- [ ] EEG
- [ ] Intracranial calcification
- [ ] Midbrain (Parinaud's) syndrome
- [ ] Normal pressure hydrocephalus
- [ ] Wernicke's encephalopathy

Spinal cord and peripheral nerve anatomy & lesions

- [ ] Innervation of specific muscles
- [ ] Median nerve/brachial plexus
- [ ] Posterior nerve root/spinal ganglia lesions
- [ ] Dorsal interosseous nerve
- [ ] Guillain-Barré
- [ ] Pyramidal tracts/posterior column pathways
- [ ] Sciatic nerve lesion
- [ ] Autonomic spondylosis
- [ ] Cervical spondylosis
- [ ] Motor neurone disease
- [ ] Paraesthesia
- [ ] Spinal cord lesions
- [ ] Polyneuropathy

Cranial nerve anatomy & lesions

- [ ] Facial nerve
- [ ] Cranial nerve lesions
- [ ] Third nerve palsy/pupillary reflex
- [ ] Bulbar palsy
- [ ] Internuclear ophthalmoplegia
- [ ] 4th nerve palsy

Dyskinesias

- [ ] Ataxia
- [ ] Benign essential tremor
- [ ] Dyskinesia
- [ ] Parkinson's disease

Muscular disorders

- [ ] Duchenne muscular dystrophy
- [ ] Myotonic dystrophy
- [ ] Myaesthenia gravis

Miscellaneous

- [ ] Multiple sclerosis
- [ ] Headache/migraine
- [ ] Lumbar puncture/CSF
- [ ] Nystagmus
- [ ] Pseudofits
- [ ] Vertigo/dysarthria
- [ ] CNS involvement in AIDS
- [ ] Eye disorders

PSYCHIATRY: REVISION CHECKLIST

Psychotic disorders
- [ ] Schizophrenia
- [ ] Depression
- [ ] Mania
- [ ] Hallucinations/delusions

Anxiety states/compulsive disorders
- [ ] Neurosis/psychogenic/conversion disorders
- [ ] Obsessional/compulsive disorders
- [ ] Panic attack

Eating disorders
- [ ] Anorexia nervosa
- [ ] Bulimia

Other cognitive disorders
- [ ] Differentiation of dementia and depression
- [ ] Acute confusional state

Miscellaneous
- [ ] Psychiatric manifestations of organic disease
- [ ] Alcohol dependency
- [ ] Insomnia
- [ ] Narcolepsy
- [ ] Endocrine causes of psychiatric disease
- [ ] Psychiatric manifestations in adolescence

INDEX

Locators refer to question number.

Basic Sciences

Index

Neurology

Index

Psychiatry

PASTEST BOOKS FOR MRCP PART 1

MRCP 1 Pocket Book Series Second Edition
Further titles in this range:

Book 1:	Cardiology, Haematology, Respiratory	*1 901198 84 7*
Book 3:	Endocrinology, Gastroenterology, Nephrology	*1 901198 94 4*
Book 4:	Clinical Pharmacology, Infectious Diseases Immunology, Rheumatology	*1 901198 98 7*

Essential Revision Notes for MRCP: Revised Edition
Philip Kalra   *1 901198 59 6*
A definitive guide to revision for the MRCP examination that offers 19 chapters of informative material necessary to gain a successful exam result.

MRCP 1 'Best of Five' Multiple Choice Revision Book
Khalid Binymin   *1 901198 57 X*
This book features subject-based chapters ensuring all topics are fully covered.

MRCP 1 300 Best of Five
Geraint Rees   *1 901198 97 9*
300 brand new 'Best of Five' questions with excellent clinical scenarios encountered in everyday hospital practice.

Essential Lists for MRCP
Stuart McPherson   *1 901198 58 8*
The lists contained in this book offer a compilation of clinical, diagnostic, investigative and prognostic features of the symptoms and diseases that cover the whole spectrum of general medicine. It is invaluable for MRCP Part 1 AND Part 2.

MRCP 1 Multiple True/False Revision Book
Philip Kalra   *1 901198 95 2*
600 multiple true/false questions in subject-based chapters and three 'test yourself' practice exams to give experience of exam fomat.

MRCP Part 1 MCQs with Key Topic Summaries: Second Edition
Paul O'Neill   *1 901198 07 3*
200 MCQs with comprehensive key topic summaries that bridge the gap between standard MCQ books and textbooks.

MCQs in Basic Medical Sciences for MRCP Part 1
Philippa Easterbrook   *1 906896 34 7*
300 exam-based MCQs focusing on basic sciences with expanded teaching notes.

PASTEST

PasTest has been established since 1972 and is the leading provider of exam-related medical revision course sand books in the UK. The company has a dedicated customer services team to ensure that doctors can easily get up to date information about our products and to ensure that their orders are dealt with efficiently. Our extensive experience means that we are always one step ahead when it comes to knowledge of the current trends and contents of the Royal College exams.

In the last 12 months we have sold over 67,000 books to medical students and qualified doctors. These may be purchased through bookshops, over the telephone or online at our website. All books are reviewed prior to publication to ensure that they mirror the needs of candidates and therefore act as an invaluable aid to exam preparation.

Test yourself online
PasTest Online is a new database that will be launched this year. With more than 1500 Best of Five questions prepared by experts, PasTest Online:

- enables you to test yourself whenever you want

- is accessible whatever time of day

- is reasonably priced and has excellent exam revision tips

- has a choice of mock exam, random questions and specialist questions. This means that you can test yourself in certain weak areas or take a mock exam.

Interested? Try a free demo at www.pastestonline.co.uk

100% Money Back Guarantee
We're sure you will find our study books invaluable, but in the unlikely event that you are not entirely happy, we will give you your money back – guaranteed.

Delivery to your Door
With a busy lifestyle, nobody enjoys walking to the shops for something that may or may not be in stock. Let us take the hassle and deliver direct to your door. We will despatch your book within 24 hours of receiving your order. We also offer free delivery on books for medical students to UK addresses.

How to Order:

🖳 www.pastest.co.uk

To order books safely and securely online, shop at our website.

☎ **Telephone: +44 (0)1565 752000**

🖶 **Fax: +44 (0)1565 650264**

✉ **PasTest Ltd, FREEPOST, Knutsford, WA16 7BR.**

WITHDRAWN